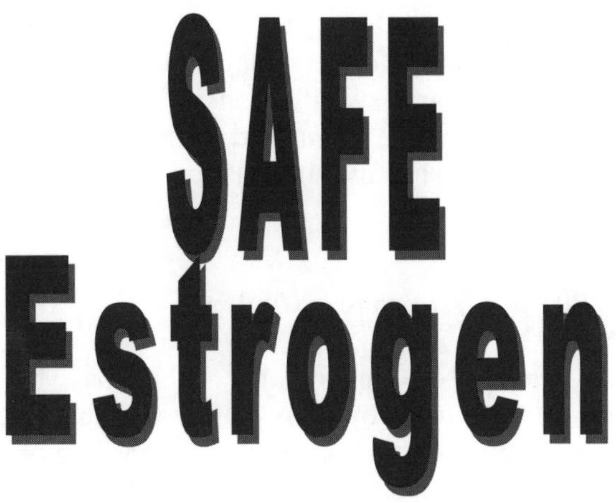

Reduce Your Breast Cancer Risk By 90%

Dr. Edward J. Conley
Assistant Clinical Professor of Medicine
Michigan State University

Vitality Press, Inc.
Flint, Michigan

This book is not intended to provide personal medical advice or treatment, nor be a substitute for personalized medical care. Never stop or begin any medical regime without consulting your physician. The publisher, author and anyone connected with this book shall not be responsible for anyone using the information contained as a self-help medical guide.

ISBN 0-9652544-2-9

Library of Congress Control Number: 2003110439

Conley, Edward J.
Safe Estrogen: Reduce Your Breast Cancer Risk by 90%/
by Dr. Edward J. Conley
Includes bibliographical references and index.
1. Breast Cancer. 2. Women's Health. 3. Health. 4. Menopause.
5. Estrogen. 6. Hormone Replacement Therapy. I. Title

Cover Design by EK Graphic Design
www.ekgraphicdesign.com

Printed in the United States

Published By
Vitality Press, Inc.
G3494 Beecher Rd
Flint, MI 48532

For Products and Information
www.SafeEstrogen.com

Table of Contents

Author and Publisher's Note

This book is a general reference guide to using estrogen and reducing breast cancer risk. The information contained is provided to the reader as a help in making informed choices about their health and healthcare.

This book is not intended to provide personal medical advice or treatment, nor be a substitute for personalized medical care. Never stop or begin any medical regime without consulting your physician. The publisher, author and anyone connected with this book shall not be responsible for anyone using the information contained as a self-help medical guide.

Every effort has been made to make this book as accurate as possible; however, there may be mistakes both typographical and in content.

Introduction

On July 17, 2002 the bubble broke. No, I am not talking about the stock market; I am speaking of the estrogen bubble. On that date, it was reported in the Journal of the American Medical Association that the Woman's Health Initiative (WHI) trial had been halted due to an "unacceptable" increase in breast cancer for women on conjugated estrogen 0.625, plus synthetic medroxyprogesterone 2.5 mg. The massive press coverage the announcement received ensured that even the pharmaceutical giants could not keep it quiet.

For at least a decade, studies had shown estrogen supplementation more than likely increased the risk of breast cancer, yet no one wanted to rock the boat. By 2000, 38% of post menopausal women in the United States used hormone replacement therapy (HRT). [1] Forty-six million prescriptions were written for Premarin (conjugated estrogens), making it the second most prescribed medication in the United States. It accounted for more than 1 billion dollars in sales per year. Another 22.3 million prescriptions were written for Prempro (conjugated estrogens plus medroxyprogesterone acetate). Doctors continued to prescribe strong estrogen supplementation because the pharmaceutical companies told them it was okay. Very few doctors were willing to stand up and take the abuse that comes along with questioning "traditional medical therapy" or with being outside the main stream. Therefore, throughout the 80's and 90's things continued status quo.

With the publication of that report and the associated news coverage, doctors could no longer ignore the risks of strong estrogen supplementation. Doctors started telling millions of women to stop the estrogen and endure the hot flashes, sleep disturbances, brain fog, sexual dysfunction, and general decrease in quality of life. The alternative was to continue the use of synthetic estrogens and risk an increase in breast cancer. What a terrible choice to see a significant reduction in your quality of life or continue on medication that reduces your symptoms but increases your risk of cancer.

Suppose there was an estrogen that controlled your menopausal symptoms without increasing your risk of breast cancer. What if, with some mild adjustments, you could reduce your risk of breast cancer by 90% while using this safer estrogen? What would this information be worth to you? This year 200,000 women in the United States will hear the dreaded words "YOU HAVE BREAST CANCER". One out of eight women get breast cancer. Eighty thousand will pay the ultimate price with their lives. The question is: Will It be You? What would you pay never to hear the words, "you have breast cancer"? What price can you put on your breasts? What price can you put on your life? What about the price of pain and suffering for you and your family even if you survive? How much would you be willing to pay to see your children and your grandchildren grow up? Of course you cannot put a price on any of these things. That is why they are called PRICELESS. Would you be willing to spend a little time and a few dollars to learn what type of estrogen does not increase the risk of breast cancer and the natural steps you can take to reduce your risk of breast cancer by as much as 90%? I bet most of you would. It seems to be a no-brainer. If only this information were available. What wonderful, life changing knowledge that would be!

Well, if you come with me for a little while, you will learn this life changing knowledge. In this book we will discuss:

- Why the estrogen you are taking increases your risk of breast cancer.
- A safer estrogen that does not increase your risk yet controls your symptoms.
- Your estrogen quotient (EQ) and why women with low EQ's have a 50% higher risk of breast cancer.
- Your EMI (estrogen metabolite index) and why women with lower EMI's have a 50% greater risk of breast cancer.
- Breast cancer causing chemicals that you eat every day and how you can block them from harming your breasts.
- Natural foods and supplements that reduce your risk of cancer.
- Natural phytonutrients you can use to control menopausal symptoms and reduce your breast cancer risk by another 50%.
- Supplements that improve your breast cancer suppression genes BRCA-1.
- Antioxidants that safeguard your breasts from damage and protect you from cancer!
- Best of all, how to combine all of the above into an easy-to-use, inexpensive program that will reduce your breast cancer risk by 90% or more.

You may be asking: "Why doesn't my doctor know this information?" This program consists of natural foods and/or supplements which cannot be patented. There is very little financial incentive for the pharmaceutical industry to do research on or to promote these products. Doctors get a large percentage of their information from the pharmaceutical industry. In addition, as strange as it may sound, doctors are not trained to keep you from getting breast cancer. Remember, doctors are trained to concentrate on fighting a "war with cancer" once you already have it.

Once you read this book you will have a far better understanding of what causes breast cancer and how to prevent it than your physician.

Lastly, our government has let us down. Our governmental agencies have been so busy protecting the pharmaceutical industry that they neglected to do the appropriate research that would have protected you. This is not surprising, since the pharmaceutical industry is a major donor to both political parties. In addition, many of the people in the governmental health agencies come from, and will return to the pharmaceutical industry. It should be said right now that the pharmaceutical industry is not evil. You must understand, however, that the pharmaceutical industry's job, as is with all industries, is to create money for shareholders. A pharmaceutical company is not there to protect you, to promote products that are cheap, or to promote products of which they do not own a patent. A good example is lowering of cholesterol. Pharmaceutical companies are interested in reducing your cholesterol levels, because they have a medication that will do so, on which they own the patent and can make significant profits. Neither you nor your doctor will hear about cheap alternatives if the pharmaceutical industry has their way.

The "war on cancer" has cost us hundreds of billions of dollars. What have we gotten for all this money? What we have received is an increasing rate of breast cancer and nearly six million women with breast cancer since 1970, (with over two million dead.) I SAY ENOUGH! I hope researchers find their "cure for cancer". In the meantime, we are going to work to keep you from getting breast cancer.

As the United States so sadly found out on September 11, 2001, an ounce of prevention is worth several tons of "cure." Remember knowledge is power. My hope is this knowledge will empower you to take control of your health and your life.

Can I offer you a fool-proof guarantee that even if you follow every recommendation in this book you will never get breast cancer? The answer is No. You must understand that this is the real world. There are no guarantees. What I can tell you is that for a few dollars and a little work, you can reduce your risk of breast cancer by up to 90%. If you do this, my sincere hope would be that you and your loved ones will never have to hear those dreaded words "YOU HAVE BREAST CANCER".

So, where do we begin? Let's start by clearing up a misconception that everyone who gets breast cancer is genetically predisposed. Then we will move on to discuss estrogen, how it works, what role it plays in breast cancer and why millions of women have been taking the type of estrogen that has increased their risk of breast cancer.

---

[1] JAMA, "Failure of Estrogen Plus Progesterone Therapy for Prevention" (17, July, 2002), Volume 288, #3.

1

Genetics: Is Breast Cancer Inherited?

Many of you have an incorrect understanding of genetics. You believed that if you have the genes for breast cancer you will get breast cancer, that it is predetermined. In addition, many of you believe that everyone that gets breast cancer has a genetic predisposition. Yet the reality is only a minority of women, who get breast cancer, have a true genetic predisposition. The majority of women who get breast cancer do not have a genetic predisposition. In fact, there was a wonderful study that sheds light on the genetic vs. environment debate. This study published in The New England Journal of Medicine in 2000 showed only approximately 27% of breast cancer is genetic. [1] This means that 73% of those studied had no genetic predisposition. How was this study done? Researchers looked at 44,788 pairs of twins from Scandinavia to evaluate the risk of cancer at 28 different sites. The results found 27% of the women who were the twin of a woman with breast cancer actually got breast cancer. This, of course, means that 73% of the twin sisters did not get breast cancer. If breast cancer is truly genetically predetermined, why didn't all of the twin sisters of those women with breast cancer also have breast cancer? The answer is breast cancer is not entirely genetically predetermined. The women who did not get breast cancer did something different than their sisters that allowed them to avoid it. So, what did they do? This we do not know, since the study did not evaluate the non-cancer twin to see what variables were different, such as diet, etc. The conclusion of the study was as follows; "Inherited genetic factors make a minor contribution to susceptibility to most types of neoplasms (cancer). This finding indicates the environment has the principal role in causing sporadic cancer." If environmental factors play a major role in causing breast cancer, why don't we know what these factors are so that we can avoid them and reduce our risk? The answer is, to a great extent, we do know these factors! The problem is there is not a lot of money to be made in keeping you from getting breast cancer. In fact, you will see that many of the changes you will make are extremely inexpensive.

Many of the supplements that you can take to reduce your risk cannot be patented. Therefore, major pharmaceutical companies are not interested. As stated before, our government has done little research on this because it is so closely tied to the pharmaceutical industry. In addition, there is a bias in the medical community against natural/nutritional preventive medicine. As we talked about in the introduction, doctors are used to battling breast cancer. Most of you would be shocked, how little training a physician receives in how to keep you from becoming ill or preventing getting cancer.

Lastly, there has been a significant amount of disinformation spread by various sources that the causes of cancer are just too intricate for us to know. The causes, supposedly, are unknowable at this time; therefore, there is nothing you can do about it, except to just sit and wait. As you will see throughout this book, that is a fallacy. I do not pretend to know each and every cause of breast cancer. Certainly, significant information will be discovered over the next decade that we do not know now. However, there has been a large amount of research conducted. Very compelling studies have been completed that show how to reduce the risk of breast cancer for most women.

Before we go on to the environmental factors, let's take some time to talk about genetic factors, since many of you have close relatives who have had breast cancer. Everyone will hear more and more about the genetic tests available that can evaluate if you have a genetic predisposition. Many of you will wonder if you should have these tests done. Furthermore, if the tests are positive, is there anything you can do about it? Let's start with what genetic tests are available and what they tell you.

<u>BRCA-1 and BRCA-2</u>

These are tumor suppressor genes, which help with DNA repair. BRCA-1 is located on chromosome 17. BRCA-2 is located on chromosome 13. There are several more tumor suppression genes that are currently under investigation, but these are the two genes whose mutations are most closely associated with an increased genetic risk of breast cancer. Inherited mutations are responsible for a minority of breast cancer, only about 7-10% of all breast cancers. Yet, if you do have one of these genetic mutations, your risk of breast cancer is significantly higher. If you have a BRCA mutation by age 50, your risk is 33-50% (significantly higher than the general population). By age 70, your risk is 55-80%. You also have a 28-44% risk of ovarian cancer by age 70-80. [4]

How does this work? Like all genes you have two copies of BRCA-1 and BRCA-2. In a "normal woman" to get a mutation you must have damage to both copies of the gene. Women with inherited mutations are born with a mutation to one copy of the BRCA-1 or BRCA-2. This means you only need to damage the other normal copy to cause a mutation. Damaging one copy of the gene, of course, is much easier than damaging two copies. A good analogy of this is, if you had two tires on each wheel, and have a flat or blowout on one tire you would still have one intact tire and can continue to drive. But our cars are built with one tire on each wheel, so a blowout of that tire causes significant instability.

Women from the general population only have about ¼ of 1% (0.25%) chance of BRCA-1 mutation. Certain ethnic groups have a significantly increased chance. An example of this is, women of Ashkenazi Jewish decent, have a 2.5-3% chance of BRCA-1 mutation. Although this is still quite low, it is 12 times higher than the general population.

How do you know if you have a BRCA-1 or BRCA-2 mutation? Testing is available through the Myriad Genetics Laboratory or through your local oncologist and geneticist.

<u>Who Should be Tested?</u>

The following are some characteristics of families with hereditary cancer syndromes:

- Several relatives with breast cancer and/or ovarian cancer.
- Unusually young age of onset of the cancers.
- Several relatives with cancer known to occur together as part of a known disorder.
- Two or more primary cancers in the same person. (Primary means that they are not metastasized from another cancer.)
- Cancers in both breasts and/or in both ovaries.
- Family history associated with autosomal dominant inheritance. [2]

If you have had several relatives with breast cancer, particularly if the cancer occurred younger than age 50, and/or family members have had breast cancer in both breasts or ovaries, you should consider getting tested for an inherited BRCA-1 or BRCA-2 mutation.

<u>What can be done if you have a genetic BRCA-1/BRCA-2 abnormality?</u>

- Very close surveillance. If you have only one intact copy of BRCA-1/BRCA-2, then you need much closer monitoring and at a younger age than a woman who does not have the mutation.

- Consider Tamoxifen or Raloxifene. One study has shown that in women with BRCA mutations who have been diagnosed with breast cancer, Tamoxifen reduced the risk of developing cancer in the other breast by 75%. (Tamoxifen was used for 2-4 years. [3] (Please see our discussion of Tamoxifen and/or Raloxifene for the associated possible side effects.)

- Prophylactic bilateral mastectomy and/or oophorectomy (removal of both breasts and ovaries). This is a recommendation that I personally disagree with, but is still an option for those of you at very high risk. Prophylactic mastectomy reduces the risk of breast cancer by 90% in women with a family history. [4] The goal of this book is to show you ways of reducing your risk of breast cancer without having your breasts removed. Later we will discuss nutritional factors that actually improve the performance of BRCA-1. This is information that traditional medicine does not know. In my opinion, the recommendation to remove both breasts prophylactically is comparable to the civil war days when a soldier had a wound to his toe, they would remove the leg to prevent gangrene.

> We are here to give you information on how to avoid breast cancer while keeping your breasts. So, what can be done if you are part of the small percentage of women with BRCA mutations? YOU MUST DO EVERYTHING YOU CAN TO PROTECT YOUR ONE NORMAL COPY OF BRCA-1 AND/OR BRCA-2. This includes taking the following supplements: 1) I3C and/or DIM. 2) Folate and B-12. 3) Curcumin. 4) Green tea phenols. 5) An aggressive antioxidant program.

We will discuss all of these nutrients in great detail in later chapters. I think you will find this information extraordinary since we will discuss one study that shows that these nutrients can protect BRCA genes from intentional damage. This is vital groundbreaking research for those of you with BRCA mutations. For the rest of you, who were not born with inherited mutations, you want to do everything possible to protect your BRCA-1 and BRCA-2 tumor suppression genes. We will also discuss how those of you with two intact BRCA genes can damage both of them through free radical oxidative damage. More important, we will discuss how you can prevent that from happening.

Summary

Genetic BRCA-1 and BRCA-2 mutations account for only 7-10% of all breast cancer. Other genetic factors account for possibly as much as 17-20%. This means that 70% of breast cancer is not directly genetically inherited, but caused by environmental factors. The majority of you were born with intact BRCA genes. What causes breast cancer is not that you were born with mutated genes, but that they became damaged throughout your lifetime. If this is the case, and studies show that it is, then 70% of you should be able to protect your tumor suppression genes and prevent yourself from getting breast cancer. Even if you have some inherited genetic susceptibility to breast cancer, there is a tremendous amount that you can do to keep your one remaining tumor suppressor gene intact. This will reduce your risk and hopefully prevent breast cancer in the future.

Now that we have briefly reviewed the genetic factors involved, we need to discuss estrogen—the role it plays in causing breast cancer and the steps you can take to prevent estrogen from harming your breasts.

---

[1] "Environmental and Heritable Factors in the Causation of Cancer" New England Journal of Medicine, Volume 343, #2 (13 July 2000).

[2] Paschold JC et al. "Hereditary Breast Cancer and Update; The Female Patient" Volume 27 (January 2002):15-24.

3 Lancet 2000; 356 (9245):1876-81.

4 "BRCA News, Summer 2001" Volume 1, Reference The New England Journal of Medicine (1999); 340:77-84.

5 The Journal of Nutrition (2000).

2

Does Estrogen Cause Breast Cancer?

Estrogen alone does not cause breast cancer. If that were true, every 18-year-old would have cancer since that is the age when your estrogen levels are highest. Breast cancer is a complex process in which many factors combine to cause, what we know and call, cancer. (Much like in the movie, The Perfect Storm™, George Clooney and his mates could have survived one or two storms, but as the movie shows, when three storms collided to make a massive typhoon, it was too much to survive.) Breast cancer is a lot like that. Genetic predisposition plays a part, although that role has been greatly exaggerated. Environmental factors play the greatest role in the causation of all cancer, particularly breast cancer. We discussed in chapter one genetic predisposition vs. environmental factors. It is important to realize that the development of breast cancer depends on several important factors:

1. How much and what type of estrogen you make.
2. Are you detoxifying estrogen to the more dangerous metabolites, which increase your risk of breast cancer?
3. Are you taking the type of estrogen supplement that increases your breast cancer risk and how long have you been taking that supplement?
4. Are you low in the essential nutrients necessary to metabolize estrogen to the "good metabolite?"
5. Do you lack the important antioxidants that are vital in repairing and protecting the DNA in your breast tissue?

6. Have you been exposed to the chemicals that mimic estrogen and cause your breast cells to reproduce wildly? (Nearly all American women have traces of these chemicals in their breast milk).

So you see, breast cancer is a far more complex issue than the relatively simple question: Does estrogen cause breast cancer? The answer to that question lies to a great degree in how you answer questions 1-6. We will review each one of these factors in detail throughout this book. You will learn how to alter each one of these risk factors, so they begin to work in your favor.

Let's take some time to talk about estrogen. There is so much information and/or misinformation concerning estrogen, that it can become confusing. We will begin talking about the different types of estrogen, (estrogen is not one hormone, but multiple hormones), and which estrogens contribute to breast cancer and which estrogen may protect against breast cancer.

3

The Three Major Types of Estrogen

Most women think of estrogen as a single hormone, when in reality it is three separate hormones: Estrone (E1), Estradiol (E2), and Estriol (E3), (See Figure 3A). Most of you have never heard of Estriol (E3), which is the type of estrogen that is highest in your body. In fact, a recent study has shown Estriol was significantly higher than the sum of Estrone (E1) and Estradiol (E2).[1] Estrone (E1) and Estradiol (E2) are the strongest estrogens you make. You produce them in lower amounts and they fluctuate more significantly than Estriol (E3). Doctors have prescribed the strong estrogens as supplements for nearly 50 years. Most doctors mistakenly thought that since Estriol (E3) was weaker, that it was too weak to be effective as replacement therapy. They believed because Estrone (E1) and Estradiol (E2) were stronger and relieved menopausal symptoms in lower dosages that they were the best estrogens to give for menopausal replacement. It now appears that this was an incorrect assumption! Estriol (E3), the weaker estrogen, is naturally high in a woman for a reason: To protect your breasts from overstimulation and overproduction of breast cells. By giving women Estrone (E1) and Estradiol (E2) as supplements, doctors decreased the Estrogen Quotient (EQ) for millions of women for half a century. The estrogen quotient (EQ) is equal to the amount of Estriol (E3) divided by Estrone (E1) plus Estradiol (E2). (See Figure 3B)

Figure 3A

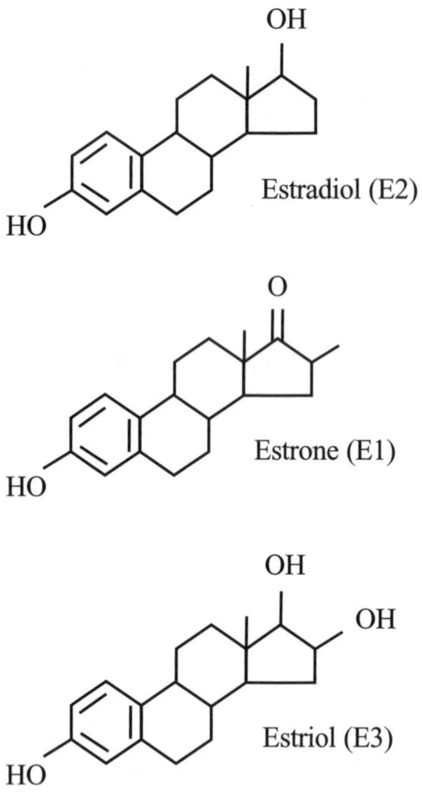

OH

HO

Estradiol (E2)

O

HO

Estrone (E1)

OH

OH

HO

Estriol (E3)

$$EQ = \frac{\text{Estriol (E3)}}{\text{Estrone (E1)} + \text{Estradiol (E2)}}$$

Figure 3B

Your EQ is one of the best predictors of your risk of breast cancer.[2] As you can see from figure 3B, when you take supplemental Estradiol (E2) or Estrone (E1) without getting increased amounts of Estriol (E3), by definition, you lower your EQ and increase your risk of breast cancer. Even worse, if you are menopausal or post-menopausal, you are making less Estriol (E3) than when you were pre-menopausal, therefore, your Estriol (E3) is lower, (in the case of surgical menopause, very low) and you are taking supplemental Estrone (E1) or Estradiol (E2). This reduces your estrogen quotient dramatically. This is a recipe for increasing your risk of breast cancer! Doctors have unknowingly been helping to create lower estrogen quotients and therefore increasing the risk of breast cancer through the very medicines they have been prescribing to control postmenopausal symptoms. To compound this problem, doctors have been prescribing these strong estrogens in the worst possible form, PILLS. Oral Estrone (E1) and Estradiol (E2) are the most commonly prescribed estrogen replacement therapy (ERT) in the world. In the year 2000, nearly 70 million prescriptions were written in the United States for Premarin and/or Prempro alone.[3] Before we discuss why the pill form is the worst possible way to take estrogen, let's review the types of estrogen and their effects on the body.

Estradiol (E2)

This is the most commonly prescribed estrogen replacement. I include in this category, conjugated estrogens, since they are converted to 17 beta-estradiol in the body. Conjugated estrogens were one of the first supplemental estrogens developed for commercial use during the 20th Century. They are made by collecting the urine from pregnant horses (mares) and refining that urine to collect the estrogen. (Remember, estrogen is not made by plants, only animals.) Although it would seem that conjugated estrogens might be safer since they are from a "natural source", this form of supplement has several possible problems.

1) Conjugated estrogens are converted to 17 beta-estradiol in the body. 17 beta-estradiol goes into the estrogen quotient as Estradiol (E2) and, by definition, lowers the estrogen quotient and increases breast cancer risk. The higher dose of conjugated estrogens you take, the lower your estrogen quotient.

2) 17 beta-estradiol is predominantly converted in your liver to the 16 OH metabolite. As we will discuss in Chapter 5, 16 OH metabolites are associated with <u>increased</u> risk of breast cancer. The higher your level of 16 OH metabolites, the higher your risk of breast cancer.

3) There are estrogens in conjugated estrogen that horses need, but women may not need, such as, Equinol.

4) Conjugated estrogens are usually prescribed in pill form. Therefore, they have a major problem associated with them, named the <u>FIRST PASS EFFECT</u>.

Estrogen supplements taken in pill form are absorbed through the digestive tract and sent to the liver to be metabolized. Up to 90% of the estrogen is metabolized in the liver prior to being released in the general circulation and sent to your tissues. This means that the majority of an estradiol supplement (pill) is metabolized in the liver to the 16 OH metabolite. It is the 16 OH metabolite that your breast tissue receives. As already mentioned, the 16 OH metabolite has been associated with an <u>increased</u> risk of breast cancer. The lower your 16 OH metabolite level, the <u>lower</u> your risk to breast cancer. So, the question is: Why in the world would you want to take an estrogen that lowers your EQ and is converted to predominantly the 16 OH metabolite, <u>which is associated with the increased breast cancer risk?</u>

How Can You Avoid the First Pass Effect?

Transdermal (through the skin) estrogen is available by patch or cream. Estrogen placed on the skin goes directly into the blood stream and is delivered to your breasts before it goes to the liver. This means that your breasts actually "see" the estrogen supplement first, not the 16 OH metabolite. It is estrogen that binds to the estrogen receptors (ER) in your breasts not the 16 OH metabolite. That is the good news.

The bad news is that most estrogen patches or creams are the strong form of estrogen, either Estradiol or conjugated estrogens. This means that they will still lower your estrogen quotient (EQ), and increase your risk of breast cancer. Even though you have improved the first pass effect, the strong estrogens lower your EQ and eventually metabolize predominantly to the 16 OH metabolite. Both of these factors will increase your risk of breast cancer. There is an estrogen cream available that does not lower your estrogen quotient. In fact, it increases your EQ and lowers your breast cancer risk.

In addition, this type of estrogen is not converted to the 16 OH metabolite. The name of this cream is Estriol (E3) and this form of estrogen will be discussed in the next chapter.

There is another problem with estrogen pills. Estrogen pills/tablets release their medicine unevenly. When you take a pill/tablet the level of estrogen in your blood goes higher in the first few hours, and lowers later in the day. Symptoms often return after a few hours, so you must take another tablet or a stronger dose the first time. This causes you to take a dose higher than you might ordinarily need if you were using a cream or patch. A cream releases more slowly, using your skin as a slow release mechanism. (The patch uses a slow release barrier.) Cream or patch, gives you a slower, steadier release of medication, plus better absorption. This allows you to use a lower dose than you would have to use with oral medication.

<u>Estrone (E1) (Ogen® Ortho-Est®)</u>

Estrone is usually given as Estrone (E1) sodium sulfate (as Estropipate). It is converted in the body, primarily to the 16 OH (bad metabolite). Estrone (E1) is predominantly given via pill, and therefore, it has all of the problems associated with strong oral estrogen replacement that we have discussed. Estrone (E1) has been linked with <u>increasing</u> the risk of breast cancer. The exact mechanism of this is unknown. We already know that taking Estrone (E1) lowers your estrogen quotient (EQ). The lower estrogen quotient <u>increases</u> your risk of breast cancer. Estrone (E1) is also predominantly converted to the 16 OH metabolite. We already know that increasing levels of 16 OH metabolites <u>increase</u> your risk of breast cancer. These are two possible explanations why Estrone (E1) can increase your overall risk of breast cancer.

<u>Why Take Estrogen in the First Place?</u>

Fourteen million women in the United States are on supplemental estrogen replacement therapy (ERT). In addition, millions of women throughout the world take estrogen replacement therapy to control estrogen deficiency symptoms caused by either natural or surgical menopause. Symptoms of estrogen deficiency include:

- <u>Classical menopausal symptoms:</u> Hot flashes, vaginal dryness, night sweats, sleep disturbances, depression, reduced libido, loss of enjoyment of sex, and increased urinary incontinence.

- <u>Cognitive decline:</u> Difficulty with short-term memory and trouble processing information.

- Osteoporosis: Estrogen replacement reduces the risks of osteoporosis by as much as 30-60%.

- Heart disease: The data is more controversial concerning ERT's ability to reduce the risk of heart disease. Some studies in the past have shown a reduction of heart disease for those women taking ERT. More recent studies, however, have questioned that conclusion. The type of estrogen and the dose given could make a significant difference in the reduction of heart disease. Estrogen traditionally has been thought to be the reason why women have a lower risk of heart attack up to menopause. After menopause, a woman's risk increases rapidly and after a few years it approaches the risk for men. Almost all of the studies on heart disease have used the strong estrogens, Estrone (E1), or Estradiol (E2) as their estrogen replacement (ERT). As we will see in the next chapter, it may not be the strong estrogens that confer the protective effect, but a different hormone or a combination of hormones.

Depending on the individual, the decrease of estrogen at menopause can range from irritating to devastating. Vaginal dryness and lack of lubrication can be frustrating, but usually helped with a water based lubricant. This problem can become severe, however, since the lack of estrogen causes the vagina to lose the ability to stretch. Many women lose enough of their elasticity that intercourse becomes intolerable. Many women develop sleep disturbances, depression, fatigue and memory disturbances, all of which can be devastating to their ability to function on a day-to-day basis. The importance of a good night's sleep cannot be overemphasized. For many women, the problem is twofold.

1) Decreased amount of sleep due to hot flashes, night sweats and other neurological factors. You may wake up many times throughout the night and have trouble getting back to sleep. If these disruptions continue for a long period of time, you are in trouble. No one can stand to have sleep disturbances for very

long without it significantly impacting their quality of life. Without sleep, we simply start breaking down. One of the first clinical signs of menopause can be sleep disruption. Prior to recognizing this, I have treated women for sleep disturbances, usually with sleep medications. After several months or years they developed hot flashes and I would place them on estrogen replacement (ERT). Magically, their sleep problems disappeared. Once I recognized this, I was alerted to the fact that sleep disturbances may be a subtle first sign of perimenopause. When I see a woman in her late 30's or 40's with sleep disturbances, I consider hormone dysfunction as a possible cause, particularly if they complained of waking up early in the morning and were not able to get back to sleep.

2) Decreased quality of sleep. Lack of estrogen significantly decreases your sleep quality along with quantity.

Summary

In this chapter we reviewed two of the three major estrogens, Estrone (E1) and Estradiol (E2). We reviewed that by definition, taking supplements of these two strong estrogens lowers your estrogen quotient (EQ) and increases your risk of breast cancer.

We found out that these estrogens are predominantly converted to the 16 OH (bad metabolites). By definition, the 16 OH metabolite decreases your estrogen metabolite index (EMI) and therefore increases your risk of breast cancer. We will discuss the EMI in detail in Chapter 5. Additionally, we discovered that most women are given the pill form of estrogen supplementation, which is predominantly transformed by the liver into metabolites prior to being released to the general circulation. This means that your breast tissue "sees" estrogen metabolites and not the estrogen itself. (Dependent on the type of metabolite, this increases your risk of breast cancer).

Topical estrogen, by cream, is the only way that I recommend taking estrogen replacement therapy (ERT).

Finally, there is an estrogen replacement named Estriol (E3) that is not converted to the 16 OH metabolite, and therefore, does not lower your EMI. It increases your estrogen quotient (EQ) by definition, therefore <u>reducing</u> your risk of breast cancer. It can be given topically by cream, avoiding the first pass effect and uses your skin as a slow release mechanism to obtain steady blood levels throughout the day. The question is, does this form of estrogen control the symptoms associated with menopause, and if so, where has it been and why don't more doctors know about it? To answer that question, see Chapter 4, where we will discuss Estriol, what it is and why it is the "safest estrogen".

---

[1] Wright JV et al., "Comparative Measurements of Serum Estrogen" Alternative Medicine Review, Volume 4, #4 (1999)

[2] Lemon HM et al., "Reduced Estriol Excretion in Patients with Breast Cancer Prior to Endocrine Therapy" JAMA (June 27, 1966) Volume 196 No 13: 112-120

[3] Fletcher SW Colditz GA, Journal of the American Medical Association (17 July 2002) Volume 288 #3:366

4

Estriol (E3): The Safer Estrogen.

What is Estriol (E3)?

Estriol is the weakest of the three major estrogens your body makes. Like the other two estrogens, Estrone (E1) and Estradiol (E2), it is made from cholesterol via several steps. (See figure 4A.) [1] It has recently been shown that you make more Estriol than the other two estrogens combined. [2] Estriol is highest, however, during pregnancy when it exerts a protective effect on both fetus and mother. After delivery, your Estriol levels never go back to the point where they were prior to pregnancy. This may explain why women who have had multiple pregnancies are at a lower risk for breast cancer than women who have never been pregnant. Estriol appears to have a protective effect on the breasts and women who have been pregnant have more Estriol. Research has shown that women who had their first baby at a young age are at a reduced risk for breast cancer. These women have higher Estriol levels at an earlier age and maintain those levels for the rest of their lives. They have had Estriols protective effect for a longer period of time, which reduces the risk of breast cancer.

Why is Estriol Protective of Breast Tissue?

Estriol is not converted to the 16 OH or 4 OH metabolite. As we will see in Chapter five, high levels of the 16 OH or 4 OH metabolites increase your risk of breast cancer. Estrone (E1) and Estradiol (E2) can be converted to the 16 OH or 4 OH metabolite. (See Figure 4B.)

Figure 4A

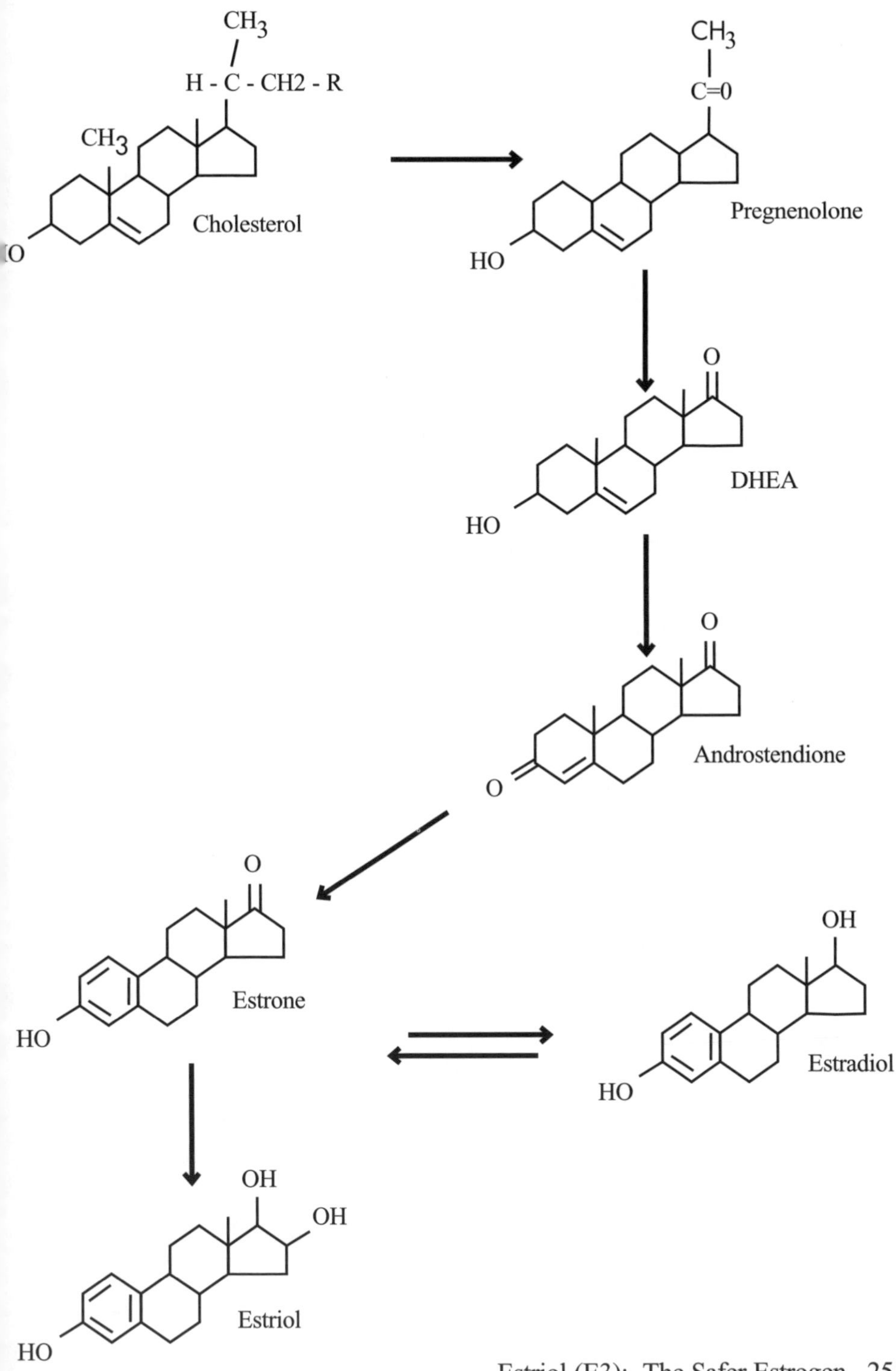

CH3
H - C - CH2 - R
CH3
Cholesterol
HO

CH3
C=0
Pregnenolone
HO

O
DHEA
HO

O
Androstendione
O

O
Estrone
HO

OH
Estradiol
HO

OH
OH
Estriol
HO

Figure 4B

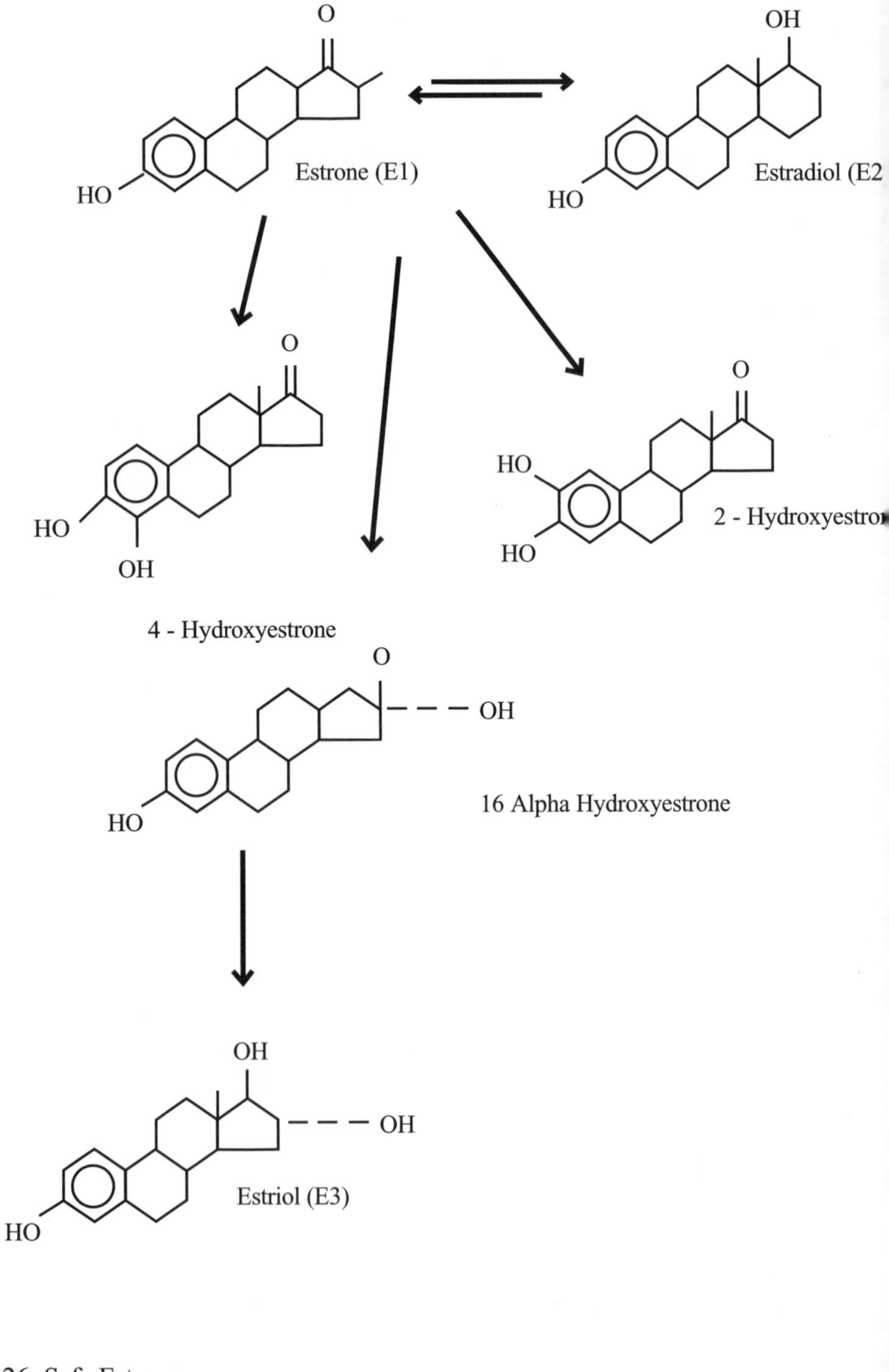

O
OH
HO
Estrone (E1)
HO
Estradiol (E2
O
O
HO
HO
OH
HO
2 - Hydroxyestro
4 - Hydroxyestrone
O
OH
HO
16 Alpha Hydroxyestrone
OH
OH
HO
Estriol (E3)

Therefore, Estriol does not lower your estrogen metabolite index (EMI). You want your EMI to be 2 or greater. When you use Estrone (E1) or Estradiol (E2) as a supplement, you lower your EMI and by definition increase your risk of breast cancer.

Estriol is a weak estrogen, but it appears to have a strong attraction for your estrogen receptors (ER). If Estriol is attached to the estrogen receptors in your breasts, the stronger estrogens like Estradiol and/or the 16 OH metabolite CAN'T bind. If the strong estrogens can't bind, they cannot overstimulate your breast tissue. Studies done on mice show that Estriol inhibits the breast cancer promoting effects of Estradiol. [3]

Another important study showed that not only did intermittent Estriol treatment not increase breast cancer, but it "demonstrated the most significant anti mammary carcinogenic activity of 22 tested compounds in rats that were fed two known carcinogens." [4] (This study was done by Dr. Henry Lemon at The University of Nebraska Medical Center. Dr. Lemon has been one of the pioneers in the study of Estriol in humans.) Remember, even though this study was done on rats, rodents are the model we use for research since you cannot give humans known carcinogens on purpose. One could argue that this is exactly what is being done to us on a massive scale, but we will discuss this in detail in our chapter on chemical carcinogens.

What are the Studies on Women?

A study done on 26 women with breast cancer showed a median estrogen quotient (EQ) of 0.5 before menopause and 0.8 after menopause. This was compared to healthy women in the study who had ratios of 1.3 before menopause and 1.2 after menopause.[5] Remember the estrogen quotient (EQ) as seen in figure 3B. This study showed that women with breast cancer had lower EQs than women who were healthy. Premenopausal women with breast cancer had EQs less than half of the healthy women, 0.5 vs 1.3. Postmenopausal women with breast cancer had EQs 44% lower than healthy post menopausal women. To have a lower EQ, by definition, you must either have less Estriol or more Estrone and/or Estradiol. We know from the study that the women with breast cancer excreted on average 30-60% less Estriol per 24 hours than the women without cancer. According to the findings of this study, the women with the higher Estriol levels, and therefore higher EQ levels, were at a significantly reduced risk of breast cancer. Why is this study and others like it so important? As you will see, Estriol is effective in reducing and/or controlling many of the symptoms of menopause including: Hot flashes, night sweats, vaginal atrophy, skin aging, cognitive decline and possibly bone loss, yet it increases the EQ, which, by definition, LOWERS your breast cancer risk.

As we will discuss, it does not seem to promote excessive uterine lining build-up or blood clots. Is it really possible that you can have your cake and eat it too? Is there really an estrogen that will control your menopausal symptoms, but not increase your breast cancer risks and MAY actually decrease your risk! Let's take a look at several studies that support this statement.

Estriol (E3) and Menopausal Symptoms.

The evidence is fairly clear that for most women Estriol (E3) can control their menopausal symptoms. The only question is, at what dosage?

- Study 1. This study done at the Medical College of Georgia used Estriol 2-8 mg per day (by mouth) on a group of 52 postmenopausal women who were having significant menopausal symptoms. The Estriol was used for six months and significant improvement was seen in hot flashes, insomnia, depression, arthralgia, headache, palpitations, dyspareunia (painful sex), vaginal dryness, and loss of libido. The most significant improvement occurred in the group that received 8 mg a day, yet improvement was seen at 4 mg per day and even 2 mg per day. (Author's Note: Remember, this Estriol was given orally. Oral Estriol is not well absorbed and may be the reason why high doses of Estriol were needed to control symptoms. If the Estriol had been given topically (through the skin), a smaller dose could have been used, since topical Estriol is better absorbed.) Of great importance is that no significant side effects were noted in any group in this study. Pap smears all remained class I (normal). Mammograms done on six women with mastoplasia showed no changes. Blood pressure and weight stayed normal. Uterine spotting occurred in only two women, but lasted for only 2-3 days and then stopped despite continued medication. Endometrial biopsies of these two women were normal. No blood clots or cardiovascular side effects were noted.[6]

- Study 2. This study was done on 20 post-menopausal women, ages 44-62. The women were given 2 mg of Estriol Succinate oral for 2 years. The authors concluded that these women had "improvement of major subjective climacteric (menopausal complaints) in 86% of patients, especially hot flashes and insomnia within three months. The atrophic genital changes caused by estrogen deficiency were improved satisfactorily.

No subjective symptoms induced by therapy were seen (side effects). Uterine bleeding was low (one patient). The study did not show, however, that Estriol could prevent osteoporosis."[7] Study 2 demonstrates that 86% of women had significant improvement, especially with hot flashes, insomnia and genital atrophy within 90 days.

- This was accomplished using 2 mg of oral Estriol and without significant side effects when monitored for two years. The only drawback for this study was that it did not show that Estriol can prevent bone loss. (We will discuss this in much greater detail later in this chapter.)
- Study 3. One hundred fifty postmenopausal women were given 1 mg of Estriol for two years. These women showed a significant improvement in their menopausal symptoms, as measured by the Kupperman index. (See Figure 4C.) On average, the Kupperman index dropped from 34 before Estriol to 6 after three months on Estriol. [8] As you can see from figure 4C, a drop in the Kupperman index from an average of 34 to an average of 6 is a significant improvement in quality of life. This change occurred on a relatively small dose of oral Estriol. (Author's Note: This is comparable to a much lower dose of topical Estriol, possibly .5 mg to 1 mg per day or less.)

These three studies show that Estriol (E3) provided women significant relief of their menopausal symptoms without signs of major side effects. Perhaps most impressive is that an oral dose as low as 1 mg gave significant relief, reducing the Kupperman index from an average of 34 pre-treatment to an average of 6 post-treatment within 90 days and no side effects were noted over the course of two years.

Kupperman Index

Symptoms "Major"	Symptoms "Minor"
• Hot flashes	• Nervousness
• Insomnia	• Dizziness
• Headache	• Joint pain
• Excessive sweating	• Tremor
• Depression	• Tachycardia
	• Irritability
	• Lack of concentration

Scale: 0 = absent

1 = present (low)

2 = moderate

3 = severe

4 = very severe

Note: Scores of "major" symptoms are doubled.

Reference: Kupperman H.S. et al., JAMA (1959); 171:1627

Figure 4C

Estriol and Your Uterus.

It is widely accepted, in the medical community, that unopposed estrogen (estrogen without progesterone), increases a woman's risk for endometrial cancer (cancer of the lining of the uterus). This increased risk is associated with the strong estrogens Estrone (E1) and Estradiol (E2). Does Estriol (E3) cause problems with over proliferation of the lining of the uterus? Let's review the medical studies.

Study 1. A meta-analysis of 12 different studies involving 214 women who used Estriol vaginal cream showed all 337 endometrial biopsies were atrophic (Not actively proliferating). Biopsies were done from 6 months to 2 years after starting Estriol. The conclusion of the meta-analysis was "single daily treatment with intravaginal Estriol in the recommended dose in post-menopausal women is safe and without an increased risk of endometrial proliferation or hyperplasia." [9]

Study 2. A study published in the Journal of the American Medical Association found no endometrial changes in 52 women given up to 8 mg of Estriol per day for 6 months. The conclusion of the authors was, "This agent (Estriol) capacity to relieve vasomotor instability (hot flashes and night sweats) and improve vaginal maturation without notable side effects are sufficient reason to include this drug in the management of post-menopausal symptoms."[10]

Study 3. A study published in the European Journal of Obstetrics and Gynecology surprisingly found that 8 mg of Estriol once per day caused slight endometrial changes, as compared with 4 mg twice a day, which caused greater endometrial changes. [11] (Author's Note: This is surprising because generally a lower dose of medication given more frequently is safer and associated with fewer side effects than a higher dose given less often. Something to consider is 8 mg a day is a high dose of Estriol and perhaps 4 mg twice per day was absorbed better and therefore delivered significantly more Estriol to the uterus than the 8 mg once per day. This is author's speculation, however, since no definite mechanism was determined in this study.)

Study 4. Estriol was given to 48 women who were scheduled for hysterectomy due to uterine prolapse. The dose was 1 mg twice daily for 10-25 days. 71% of these women showed endometrial hyperplastic changes. (Author's Note: The lining of the uterus was growing.) It should be noted that 22 of the women also received the stronger conjugated estrogen by vaginal suppository. (Author's Note: The authors of this study state no statistical significance was seen between the two groups, Estriol alone vs Estriol plus conjugated estrogens.)[12]

Discussion.

What conclusions can we draw from these studies?

- Estriol in most studies does not cause uterine endometrial hyperplasia (excessive growth of the uterine lining). In some women, it may cause proliferation if given in a large dose over a long period of time. Remember, you are a unique individual with unique biochemical responses to any medication or supplement.

- It appears to be safer to use the smallest amount of Estriol as infrequently as possible to control menopausal symptoms. Once per day appears better than twice per day. Every other day appears safer than daily. Therefore, you should use the least amount of Estriol necessary to control your symptoms.

- As we will discuss in the progesterone chapter, we almost always will use bioidentical progesterone cream in combination with Estriol. This means that rarely will Estriol be unopposed and therefore this should make the endometrial hyperplasia issue a mute point since progesterone should protect your uterus lining from overproduction and therefore prevent the small likelihood of uterine lining overgrowth with Estriol.

Estriol and Your Bones

One of the major "drawbacks" of Estriol has been that most physicians concluded that it does not protect you from osteoporosis. This is one of the reasons that the stronger estrogens "won" the confidence of the physicians and became some of the most widely prescribed medications in the world. (Author's Note: The other reason, of course, is money. The stronger estrogens could be patented and become the property of pharmaceutical corporations. Estriol, because it is a natural substance, could not be patented and therefore was not promoted.)

Is the "Knock" on Estriol Justified? Does It Protect You From Osteoporosis? Let's look at the scientific studies.

Study 1. A study done in Japan showed an increase in bone mineral density (BMD) after 2 mg a day of Estriol plus 800 mg of calcium lactate for almost a year (50 weeks). BMD increased 1.8%[13]

Study 2. Another Japanese study showed a small group of women (17) given Estradiol 2 mg a day, plus calcium lactate 2000 mg a day, showed an improvement in bone mineral density (BMD) of 1.7% vs a controlled group which received the calcium only. The control group actually had a decrease in BMD after 52 weeks. In addition, the Estriol group had a decrease in all measures of bone destruction vs the control group.[14]

Study 3. A third Japanese study showed 18 women given Estriol plus calcium lactate (2 mg a day of Estriol plus 1 gm a day of calcium lactate) showed an increase in bone mineral density of 5.6% with the women who just received calcium losing bone density by 4%.[15] Other studies done with Estriol have not shown improvement in bone mineral density.

Study 4. A study from the Chinese Medical Journal showed Estriol was a very effective treatment for post-menopausal symptoms, but it did not prevent osteoporosis. (As measured by quantitative computed tomography (QCT) after 1 and 2 years.)[7]

Study 5. Perhaps the most interesting study of this group is from The Institute of Obstetrics and Gynecology in Cagliari, Italy. It was reported in the Journal of Climacteric and Post-Menopause in 1996. This study showed intravaginal Estriol given to 214 healthy, post-menopausal women reduced the decrease in bone mineral density seen in the controlled group, which was given calcium only. Estriol also reduced the urinary excretion of hydroxyproline (a measure of bone loss) and slowed, but did not totally prevent the drop in bone mineral density seen with the control group. When salmon calcitonin was added to Estriol plus calcium, there was a significant improvement in bone mineral density (BMD), along with control of postmenopausal symptoms.[16] Salmon calcitonin is a medication given by injection or nasal spray as a treatment for osteopenia and/or osteoporosis. It is generally well tolerated and has few side effects. The only contradiction being, you cannot take this medication if you are allergic to salmon.

Discussion

The answer to this question is unclear. Does Estriol protect your bones from osteoporosis? Some studies say it does and others disagree. My question is, "Does it really matter?" Of course, we all agree that osteoporosis is a very serious disease that kills thousands of women per year in the United States, (including my mother). It is vital that your bones be protected. We have seen that Estriol controls menopausal symptoms with very few side effects and that it may protect bone, even without the addition of other medications. If we assume that it does not, then you can very easily maintain your bone strength by exercise, calcium supplementation, phytonutrients, natural progesterone and/or the addition of salmon calcitonin. You can use any combination of the above to maintain your bone mineral density. Monitor your bone density yearly by dual photon densitometry and urinary bone breakdown products. (For discussion on how to get the urinary bone loss breakdown product measured, see products section at the end of this book.)

Estriol and Vaginal/Urinary Complaints.

So far we have learned that Estriol does control menopausal symptoms without apparent serious side effects and that it does not appear to stimulate overgrowth of the uterus lining. The question remains, does it protect bone? Even if it does not, your bone strength can be maintained with the addition of salmon calcitonin and/or progesterone, both of which are very safe and well tolerated. Does Estriol improve vaginal function and/or poor urinary control that is associated with postmenopausal loss of estrogen? Let's look at the data.

Study 1. Estriol was given to 263 menopausal women, with half of them receiving 2-4 mg per week. This study showed that even this low dose of Estriol was able to restore normal vaginal function without causing excessive uterine endometrial growth.[17]

Study 2. This study was done on 41 women with severe atrophic vaginitis using low dose Estriol at 0.5 mg per day. "Estriol restored vaginal function and normal urethra cells with two weeks of therapy."[18] (Author's Note: Atrophic vaginitis is dysfunction of the vagina caused by lack of estrogen. Without estrogen, the lining of the vagina loses its stretchability and often becomes inflamed, red and painful. Urethral cells are the cells of the tube that carries urine from the bladder to the outside. Without estrogen, these cells can become damaged and/or distressed causing loss of urinary control, burning and/or frequency.)

Study 3. 3.5 mg of Estriol was given intravaginally for 3 months to 135 post-menopausal women with inability to hold their urine. This study showed 63% of the women improved their incontinence. Painful urination improved in all of the Estriol groups. The frequency with which the women urinated improved significantly.[19] (This study was reported in the New England Journal of Medicine.)

Study 4. Estriol was shown to improve the good bacteria in the vagina and reduce urinary tract infections. This study concluded that "intravaginal Estriol was associated with a significant decrease in vaginal pH. (Author's Note: Improved vaginal acid base balance and increased vaginal colonization with lactobacilli (good bacteria). It decreased vaginal colonization with enterobacteria (bacteria that can cause infection). These changes in colonizing microorganisms undoubtedly have a critical role in altering the susceptibility of post-menopausal women to urinary tract infection."[20]

Discussion

Estriol helps lower the pH of the vagina to a more healthy acidity, which allows better growth of good bacteria and slows the growth of bad bacteria. If the vagina stays clear of bad bacteria, there will be less urinary tract infections (UTI). The fewer UTI's the less antibiotics you need. The less antibiotics, the less damage done to the good bacteria in your vagina. (Author's Note: One of the first things most of you have discovered, when you take an antibiotic, is that you develop vaginal yeast. The reason for this is that the antibiotic kills many of the good bacteria in your vagina, but does not kill yeast or certain bad bacteria. This allows those bad bacteria and/or yeast to overgrow and cause an infection.) In addition, Estriol directly improved vaginal function and urethral cellular health. Therefore, women in these studies had less pain with intercourse, less vaginal infections, less frequency of urine, less urinary tract infections and better sexual function.

Estriol and Your Skin.

One complaint most post-menopausal women have is sagging skin! Increasing wrinkles, drooping skin of the neck, arms, tush, belly, and breasts. This is due to the fact that estrogen plays a key role in maintaining the elastin fibers in your skin. As your estrogen level drops, the skin loses its elasticity and skin wrinkles and/or sags. The result of estrogen on skin is dramatic. I have seen old wrinkled men who were placed on estrogen as a treatment for prostate cancer develop the skin of a 30-year-old in a matter of months. It is fairly well documented that strong estrogen replacement therapy (ERT) can improve your skin's elasticity, but it increases your risk of breast cancer. What about Estriol? Can it help your skin? We already have seen the risk of developing breast cancer from Estriol appear to be very low. Let's look at a couple of interesting studies that review Estriols effect on your skin.

Study 1. This study showed that Estriol at 1 mg applied once daily improved the elastin in 50% of the women treated after only 3 weeks. None of the control group improved.[21]

Study 2. From the International Journal of Dermatology, this study compared 0.3% Estriol to 0.01% Estradiol cream applied to the face and neck for 3 months. Both groups were post-menopausal women, not on other hormone replacement therapy. The conclusion was "both types of estrogen markedly improved elasticity and firmness of the skin and reduced wrinkle depth and pore size dramatically, by approximately 61-100%. In addition, skin moisture improved and no systemic hormonal side effects were noted."[22]

Discussion

Both of these studies showed that Estriol can help skin aging by improvement of elastin, collagen and moisture of the skin. It should be noted that in both of these studies, Estriol was applied directly to the skin that was measured. It is unknown how much systemic Estriol will help the face, etc. when it is applied elsewhere. My clinical judgment would be that you should see some improvement or better maintenance of your skin tone, but perhaps not as much improvement i.e. the 61-100% that was noted by direct application of the Estriol to the face.

Estriol and Cholesterol/ Blood Pressure/ Blood Clots.

Past studies have suggested that traditional ERT, (Estrone and/or Estradiol) provided some cardiac protective effect for women. Premenopausal women are at a significantly reduced risk for coronary artery disease (plugging of the heart arteries) compared with men their age. The explanation for this has always been that estrogen is the reason for the protective affect. Women on average have higher levels of "good cholesterol" (HDL) compared with men their age. HDL serves a protective effect on the arteries. After menopause cardiac lipids change, and a woman's cardiac risk climbs quickly to where within several years after menopause you are at nearly the same risk as a man your age. Recently, The Woman's Health Initiative (WHI) showed that conjugated estrogen plus synthetic progestin actually increased cardiac risk! (Author's Note: This is the study that caused so much controversy in the summer of 2002. It was stopped due to the unacceptable increase in risk of breast cancer for those women on conjugated estrogen plus synthetic progestin. However, the levels of increasing cardiac risk were nearly approaching the point where the study would be stopped for those reasons as well.)

What do the studies tell us concerning Estriol (E3)? Does it control coronary risk factors, blood pressure, and/or blood clots? Let's look at the literature.

Study 1. A study in the British Journal of Obstetrics and Gynecology showed Estriol succinate had less potential to cause blood clots than synthetic estrogen over 12 months of therapy. They found "no significant changes in concentration of plasma coagulation factors."[23]

Study 2. A Japanese study showed that Estriol at 2 mg per day improved HDL's, decreased triglycerides and total cholesterol and therefore produced a "significant improvement in overall cardiac risk profile". This improvement occurred in women aged 70-84. Interestingly, Estriol did not improve the cardiac risk profile of the younger group in the study.[24]

Study 3. A Chinese study used a synthetic long-acting form of Estriol called Nylestriol and found no increase in cardiac lipids and an improvement in HDL's (good cholesterol).[25]

Discussion

None of the studies reviewed by this author showed any adverse cardiac or clotting effects in response to Estriol use. Two small studies suggest possible improvement of cardiac risk factors with Estriol, but these studies were very small and few in number. (Author's Note: Of course a large scale study would be helpful in clarifying this matter.) At worst, however, Estriol would be cardiac neutral with signs of lower risk for blood clots as noted in the study from The British Journal of Obstetrics and Gynecology. Given the recent results of the Women's Health Initiative (WHI), showing conjugated estrogen plus synthetic progestin increased cardiac risk, increased breast cancer risk and that Estriol appears to be, at worst, cardiac neutral and, at best, mildly cardiac protective, Estriol appears to be the more reasonable supplement. In addition, Estriol improved post-menopausal symptoms without increasing breast cancer risk and with significantly less risk for blood clots.

Summary

- Estriol has been shown to improve the symptoms of menopause including hot flashes, night sweats, insomnia, depression, headache, palpitations, vaginal dryness, urinary incontinence, and loss of libido. It does so without overstimulation of breast tissue and therefore reduced risk of breast cancer as compared with the stronger estrogens Estrone (E1) and/or Estradiol (E2). Studies have shown that women with breast cancer had lower estrogen quotients (EQ) than healthy women and this lower EQ was due to lower amounts of Estriol. The women with breast cancer had Estriol levels on average 30-60% lower than the healthy women. We have discussed that higher levels of Estriol appear to be the reason why women who have had babies at a young age have a lower risk of breast cancer than women who became pregnant later in life or who have never been pregnant. In addition, we reviewed animal studies that showed Estriol was able to block breast cancer due to two strong carcinogens, better than 22 other compounds that were tested.

- Estriol does not strongly encourage uterine lining proliferation and in several studies did not increase uterine lining at all. For the sake of safety, let's assume that Estriol did mildly increase uterine proliferation; this can be very easily offset by the addition of natural bioidentical progesterone cream.

- Estriol reduces vaginal atrophy and urinary tract infections through direct improvement of vaginal cells, and secondary improvement of vaginal pH and lactobacillus (good bacteria). Estriol also has been shown to have direct improvement in the health of urethral cells (urine tube).

- Estriol does not protect bone density as well as the strong estrogens, yet when you combine it with natural progesterone and/or salmon calcitonin you get safer control of post-menopausal symptoms plus improvement in bone mineral density (BMD).

- Estriol improves skin elastin and collagen when applied directly to the skin. More than likely it improves skin elasticity better than no estrogen supplementation at all.

- Estriol appears to be cardiac neutral at worst, and possibly mildly cardio protective, although more studies need to be done to definitively show Estriols effect on cardiac lipids. It does not appear to increase the risk of blood clots (in any of the literature reviewed by this author), as opposed to the stronger estrogens Estrone (E1) and/or Estradiol (E2), both of which have increase risk of blood clots listed as known side effects.

Conclusion

Estriol (E3) is the weakest estrogen that reduces post-menopausal symptoms. It is associated with significantly lower risks of breast and uterine cancer than the stronger estrogens Estrone (E1) and/or Estradiol (E2). Estriol is excellent for the treatment of vaginal or urinary problems related to menopause and achieves improvement at very low doses. The major "knock" on Estriol is that it does not protect your bones as well as Estrone (E1) and/or Estradiol (E2). This appears to be true, yet can be compensated very easily by the addition of natural progesterone and/or salmon calcitonin. It should be noted that Estriol does protect from bone loss much better than no estrogen at all. We will discuss in the progesterone chapter that natural bioidentical progesterone improves your ability to make bone. The addition of natural progesterone to your Estriol cream may have the dual action of improving how you make bone and stabilizing and/or preventing the loss of bone. Estriol combined with the program of breast cancer prevention, as outlined in this book, should allow post-menopausal women to receive the benefits of ERT, reducing symptoms, with a subsequent dramatic improvement in quality of life and keep the possibility of dangerous life-threatening side effects, like breast cancer, to a minimum. Earlier I asked, "Can you have your estrogen and be safe too?" This chapter has shown that most women can take Estriol for control of their post-menopausal symptoms and actually reduce their risk of breast cancer by up to 90% by following the steps we will discuss in the following chapters.

Can I give you an iron clad guarantee that Estriol at any dose will never increase the risk of breast and/or uterus cancer for you? The answer is, "No". As we discussed before, all of you are unique individuals. Estriol still acts as an estrogen, and at high doses the possibility remains that it could increase your risk of cancer by overstimulating your breast tissue. What we have done in this chapter is outline a program of safer estrogen replacement therapy (ERT) using Estriol, which I hope will benefit millions of women whose symptoms are not controlled with other supplements and/or phyto nutrients. As we will discuss throughout this book, my recommendation is trial of diet and/or phyto nutrient supplementation first, then if your symptoms cannot be controlled, a trial of low-dose Estriol cream would be reasonable. If you go on Estriol therapy, you should continue to have close surveillance including, breast checks, mammograms, and Pap smears (uterine ultrasounds and/or biopsies, if indicated). For those of you on low-dose strong estrogen replacement (i.e. Estrone (E1), Estradiol (E2) or conjugated estrogens), a slow taper with changes in your diet and possibly the addition of a phyto nutrient supplement would be in order. (Authors Note: Only attempt this under a doctor's supervision. The doctor you use must be familiar with natural therapies, phytonutrients and Estriol.) For those of you on high dose estrogen replacement at 1.25 mg and above, a switch to Estriol should be strongly considered. Remember, Estriol is not as strong as Estrone, Estradiol, or conjugated estrogens, so you may have to start at 2.5 to 5 mg per day of Estriol cream for symptom control. In a few months, if your symptoms have been well controlled, you can try slowly titrating down with the supervision of your physician.

For the millions of you who have stopped all estrogen replacement therapy (ERT) due to the fear generated by the Women's Health Initiative (WHI) and are living in misery, there is a way to restore your quality of life with lower risks than your old ERT. If you stopped your ERT and are having mild symptoms, try changing your diet and/or if that does not work consider adding a phyto nutrient supplement. (See Chapter 7, Phytonutrients.) If diet changes and natural phytonutrients do not control your symptoms, then the addition of low dose Estriol could be considered. Continuing dietary changes and phyto- nutrients will help you to stay on the lowest level of Estriol possible.

What If You Already had Breast Cancer?

This is a more difficult decision. If you are currently on conjugated estrogens, Estrone and/or Estradiol, my opinion is you should switch to Estriol. In my opinion, Estriol represents a far safer supplement for you than the stronger estrogens mentioned above. Many of you are not on any replacement, and millions of you are miserable. The place to begin is with your diet. (See Chapter 7, Phytonutrients). If your quality of life is still poor with diet changes, consider a phyto nutrient supplement since these are the weakest forms of "natural estrogen supplementation". (As we have already noted, plants do not make estrogen, but these substances resemble estrogen and will help relieve some of your symptoms.) As you will see from the phyto nutrient chapter, most studies suggest phyto nutrient supplements are associated with lower risk of breast cancer, not increased risk. Remember there are no absolute iron clad guarantees. What we can say is that phytonutrient supplementation seems to be lower in risk than any estrogen supplementation.

Finally, if you need estrogen replacement to maintain a reasonable quality of life, then in my opinion Estriol is by far the safest choice. (Author's Note: I have seen one study done with Estriol in women with breast cancer. The study showed a 37% positive remission or arrest of metastatic lesions with Estriol supplementation.)[26] This is a fascinating study showing that not only does Estriol not increase the risk of breast cancer, but that it may be a cancer therapy. This is only one small study, and therefore the use of ERT in someone who has had a previous breast cancer should be a last resort. It is always an extremely difficult question for both you and your doctor: Whether to use ERT if you had a previous breast cancer. Most doctors will say "No", and I would agree. Most doctors will try selective estrogen receptor modulators (SERM) including Tamoxifen and Raloxifene.

If you have had a previous breast cancer, estrogen supplementation should be avoided. If, however, you are on ERT currently, in my opinion, you should switch to Estriol. If you are miserable and your quality of life is terrible and you have not been able to maintain control of symptoms with any other treatment, then you should discuss with your health care practitioner and/or oncologist, the possibility of Estriol, but it should always be a last resort.

So, Why Doesn't Every Doctor Know about Estriol?

In the beginning when estrogen was first discovered, it was felt that Estriol was too weak to be of any consequence. Therefore, it was ignored. Around mid century it was used as an estrogen replacement in Europe. Slowly studies were done that showed its usefulness and its safety. These studies were conducted mostly in Europe. The European studies were mostly ignored in the United States due to two reasons, 1) Estriol did not appear to protect bone as well as other estrogen replacement therapies and bone protection was a very "hot item" in the 1970's. 2) Money. Most doctors in the U.S. get their information from pharmaceutical companies, either directly or indirectly. They receive information directly through studies done and funded by the pharmaceutical corporations and indirectly through studies done at major universities. Most are funded by the pharmaceutical industry and/or governmental entities. As we have reviewed, the U.S. governmental agencies have been very close and very protective of the pharmaceutical industry. Estriol cannot be patented; therefore, no company stands to gain billions of dollars by investing the millions of dollars it costs to do extensive studies. Conjugated estrogens, Estrone and Estradiol, all could be patented, and pharmaceutical companies could and did do extensive studies on these ERTs with the results of billions of dollars in profits from their use. The only ones who could have provided women with the vital information concerning Estriol either did not know about it or did not want to know about it. Doctors were told that the strong ERTs were the treatment of choice, and very few questioned whether or not this was true. Even in the last two decades, when it started to become clear that strong ERT increased the risk of breast cancer, doctors still wanted to believe what they were being told and most did not question if there were safer alternative treatments available. This is a shame, since Estriol had been safely used in Europe for nearly half a century. (Author's Note: There is a real bias; one could say arrogance, to United States medicine. In general, American doctors dismiss European studies even when those studies are well done and published in peer review European Journals. If doctors throughout the 1980's and 90's would have paid more attention to the European studies and less attention to the misinformation they were being spoon fed, Estriol may have become the treatment of choice. This brings out one further problem with medicine in the United States and that is, doctors are selected NOT to think independently. The doctors who do best in medical school and/or residency are those who take the information they are given and utilize it without question. So, even though physicians on the whole are extremely intelligent, they are selected and taught not to question authority. No doctor would purposely harm a patient, just like no stock broker would purposely try to give you a stock tip that lost money. Yet by blindly accepting the information that they were given, doctors have unknowingly contributed to the breast cancer "epidemic" that has developed in the latter half of the 20th century.

Dose of Estriol—You and your physician should consider the following:

1) Begin with 0.5 mg Estriol cream every other day. If menopausal symptoms continue, increase slowly up to between 2-5 mg every other day, dependent on response. If not controlled on an every other day treatment regimen, may increase to daily. Every 3-6 months try to slightly reduce your dose to see if it is tolerated. If symptoms return, obviously, you can return back to your previous dose.

2) Topical Estriol is absorbed 20 times more effectively than oral (pill form). Therefore, always use topical (cream).

3) If vaginal atrophy and urinary problems are your major complaints, Estriol cream can be compounded in a vaginal form.

4) If you are unable to control your symptoms at 5 mg of Estriol daily, combination products are available, which consist of 80% Estriol, 20% Estradiol. (Example: If 1.25 mg is prescribed per day, 1 mg is Estriol and .25 mg is Estradiol. This combination is stronger than Estriol and should help to

control symptoms not controlled by pure Estriol. Remember, the stronger the estrogen, the higher the risks of side effects and/or breast cancer. It is thought, however, with the majority of this cream being Estriol; the Estriol will bind to the estrogen receptors in your breasts and help protect them against the stronger Estradiol.

5) Never use oral estrogen replacement.
6) Do not use Estriol if you are pregnant or breast feeding.
7) Do not use Estriol if you have had previous breast or ovarian cancer.
8) Use only professionally formulated topical or vaginal creams.
9) Reduce or discontinue Estriol if you develop severe breast tenderness, increased breast fibrocysts or excessive vaginal bleeding.

10) Balance Estriol with bioidentical progesterone cream. The progesterone can be placed in the same cream with the Estriol. See Chapter 9.

11) Always use the lowest dose that relieves symptoms and try small reductions in your dose every six months.

12) Work with a physician that understands Estriol therapy. Most physicians will be ignorant of what you are trying to tell them and most physicians are very resistant to taking suggestions from patients. Finding the right physician may take a little work, but it will be well worth the effort!
13) Every woman is unique. Therefore, your dose will be different than anyone else. Your response to the medication and/or side effects will be on an individual basis. The time for one-size-fits-all treatments, I hope, is coming to an end. It is vital that you work with a physician or health care practitioner that understands these principles.

14) Read the rest of this book!

Let's go on to talk about the estrogen metabolite index (EMI). As you will see, it is not just the type of estrogen you take and/or make, but how you detoxify it that determines your breast cancer risk. Let's review what the two predominant estrogen metabolites are and how one metabolite, the 2 OH can protect your breasts, while the other metabolite, 16 OH, significantly <u>increases</u> your risk of getting breast cancer.

---

[1] Lehninger; Textbook of Biochemistry: pp. 681.
[2] Wright JV, et. al.; Comparative Measurements of Serum Estriol, Estradiol, and Estrone in Non-Pregnant, Premenopausal, Woman Alternative Medicine Review, Volume ______, 1999: pp. 266-70
[3]
[4] Lemon H.M.; Pathophysiologic Consideration in the Treatment of Menopausal Patients with Estrogen; The Role of Estriol and the Prevention of Mammary Carcinoma, ACTA Endocrinol Supplemental, 1980, 233: S17-27.
[5] Lemon, H.M., et. al.; Journal of the American Medical Association; Reduced Estriol Excretion in Patients with Breast Cancer Prior to Endocrine Therapy, Volume 196 #13, 1966: pp. 1128-36.
[6] Tzingounisbava, et. al.; Estriol and the Management of the Menopause, Journal of the American Medical Association, 421, 1978, Volume 239 #16: pp. 1638-41.
[7] Yangts, et. al.; Efficacy and Safety of Estriol Replacement Therapy for Climacteric Women, Chinese Medical Journal, 1995; 55: 386-91.
[8] Perovic D., et. al.; Treatment of Climacteric Complaints with Estriol; Arzneimittelforschung, 1997; 25: pp. 962-64.
[9] Vooijs G.P. et. al.; Review of the Endometrial Safety During Intravaginal Treatment with Estriol, European Journal of Obstetrics and Gynecology and Reproduction Biology, 62, 1995: pp. 101-106.
[10] Tzinogounis B.A., et. al.; Estriol in the Management of the Menopause. Journal of the American Medical Association; April 21, 1978, 239 (16): pp. 1638-41.
[11] Punnonen R. et. al.; The Effect of Oral Estriol Succinate Therapy on the Endometrial Morphology in Post-Menopausal Women, European Journal of Obstetrics and Gynecology Reproductive Biology, 1983; 14: pp. 217-24.
[12] Montoneri C. et. al.; Effects of Estriol Administration on Human Post-Menopausal Endometrium, Clin Exp Obstetrics and Gynecology, 1987; 14: pp. 178-81.
[13] Minaguchih, et. al.; The Effects of Estriol on Bone Loss in Post-Menopausal Japanese Women, J. Obstet. Gyn. Res. 1996; 22: 259-65.

[14] Mozakim, et. al.; Usefulness of Estriol for the Treatment of Bone Loss in Post-Menopausal Women, Nippon Sanka Fiyinka Gakkai Zasshi 1996; 48: pp. 83-88. Alternative Medicine Review, Volume 3 #2 1998, pp. 105.

[15] Nishibe A., et. al.; Effects of Estriol in Bone Mineral Denisty of the Lumbar Vertebrae, Nippon Ronen Igakkai Zasshi 1996; 33: pp. 353-59. Alternative Medicine Review, Volume 3 # 2 1998; pp. 105.

[16] Melis G. B., et. al.; Salmon Calcitonin Plus Intravaginal Estriol: An Effective Treatment for the Menopause., Maturetas 24 (1996) pp. 83-90.

[17] Hustin J., et. al.; Cytological Evaluation of the Effect of Various Estrogens Given in Menopause.: ACTA Cytologica, 1977; 21: 225-28.

[18] Heimer G. M., Estriol in the Menopause, ACTA Obstet Gynecol Scand, 1987; 139: S 1-23.

[19] Schar G. et. al.: Effective Vaginal Estrogen Therapy on Urinary Incontinence in Post-Menopause, Zentrabbl Gynakol, 1995; 117: pp. 77-80.

[20] Razr, et. al.; A Controlled Trial of Intravaginal Estriol in Post-Menopausal Women with Recurrent Urinary Tract Infections, New England Journal of Medicine, 1993; 753-56.

[21] Punnonen R., et. al.; Local Estriol Treatment Improves the Structure of Elastin Fibers in the Skin of Post-Menopausal Women, Ann Chir Gynaecol 76, Supplemental 202, pp. 39-41, 1987.

[22] Schmidt J.B., et. al.; Treatment of Skin Aging with Topical Estrogens, International Journal of Dermatology, Volume 35 #9, September 1996.

[23] Toy J.L., The Effects of Long-term therapy with Estriol Succinate on the Hemostatic Mechanism in Post-Menopausal Women, British Journal of Obstetrics and Gynecology, May 1978, Volume 85, pp. 363-66.

[24] Head K.A., Estriol: Safety and Efficacy, Alternative Medicine Review, Volume 3 #2, 1998.

[25] Guo-jun C., et. al.; Nystriol Replacement Therapy in Post-Menopausal Women, Chinese Medical Journal, 1993; 106: pp. 911-16.

[26] Follingstad A.H.: Estriol, The forgotten Estrogen? JAMA, January 2, 1978, Volume 239 #1; pp. 29.

5

The Estrogen Metabolites Index (EMI)

All estrogen, regardless if produced naturally or given as a prescription, gets broken down in your liver via an enzyme system named the p-450 pathway. This p-450 system detoxifies many substances, including hormones, medicines and toxins. The detoxification of estrogen occurs along two major pathways (See figure 5A.)

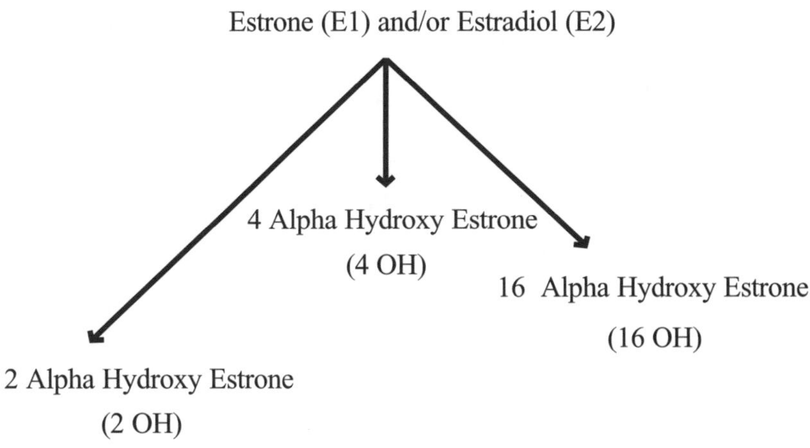

Figure 5A

The strong estrogens, Estrone (E1) and Estradiol (E2) are converted to 3 distinct types of metabolites. These include the 2 OH, 4 OH and 16 OH. No woman converts down one pathway alone. You convert a portion of your estrogen down each pathway. The important question is, how much estrogen do you convert down the 2 OH pathway (which lowers your breast cancer risk), versus the 16 OH pathway, (which increases your risk)? We will discuss these metabolites in great detail. You may ask, "Why do you have to detoxify estrogen in the first place?" If estrogen was not detoxified (metabolized), it would quickly build up in your system and overstimulate all the tissues that are sensitive to it. These include breasts, ovaries, uterus, brain, etc. This overstimulation would rapidly lead to significant symptoms, including heavy bleeding, fibrocystic breast disease, and breast cancer. It is vital for the body to maintain a balance of estrogen, not too much, not too little. (Author's Note: This is true for nearly everything in nature, and certainly for all hormones.) The majority of your estrogen follows two major pathways. The 16 OH metabolite retains significant estrogen activity. In fact, many researchers feel it is actually more potent and more dangerous than estrogen itself! Studies have shown that overproduction of 16 OH significantly increases your risk of breast cancer. The 2 OH pathway, however, has been associated with a LOWER risk of breast cancer. Low levels of 2 OH have been associated with breast cancer[1], and uterine cancer[2] (also, cervical cancer[3], and lupus[4]). Medical studies have shown that the lower your 2 OH/16 OH ratio, especially if it is below 2, the HIGHER your risk of breast cancer. What is the optimal 2 OH/16 OH ratio? No one knows the answer to this question. What we do know is that research has shown the closer your 2 OH/16 OH ratio (EMI) is to 2, the less your risk of breast cancer. The closer your ratio is to 1, the greater your risk. So the answer to my question appears to be 2 OH ÷ 16 OH = 2 or above. (Author's Note: For clarification, the 2 OH ÷ 16 OH ratio is named the estrogen metabolite index (EMI). Therefore your EMI should be 2 or above. So that you do not become confused, throughout this chapter I may refer to it as the EMI or the 2 OH ÷ 16 OH ratio. Either way it is referring to the same ratio. (See Figure 5B)

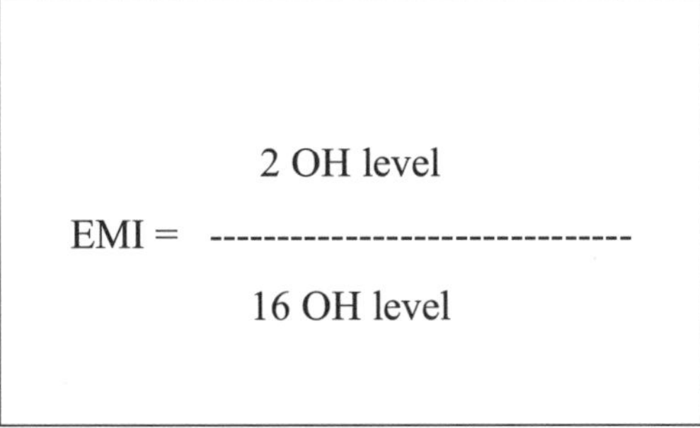

Figure 5B

<u>Study 1.</u> A large study done on women 35 and older showed that post-menopausal women who went on to develop breast cancer had a 2 OH/16 OH ratio (EMI) 15% lower than those women without breast cancer.[5] The women in the highest 1/3 of the 2 OH/16 OH ratio (EMI) had a <u>30% lower risk of developing breast cancer</u> than those in the lower 2/3. <u>Important Point:</u> this study shows that if you maintain your 2 OH/16 OH ratio (EMI) in the highest 1/3, you reduce your risk of breast cancer by 30%. This study also showed that <u>women that maintained their ratio closer to 2 had a significantly reduced breast cancer risk compared to those with ratios of 1.5!</u>

<u>Study 2.</u> Another study showed that the 2 OH/16 OH ratio <u>(EMI) was the most significant predictive factor</u> of breast cancer in post-menopausal women.[6]

<u>Study 3.</u> In postmenopausal women with breast cancer, the 2 OH/16 OH ratio (EMI) was 1.4 vs matched controls (women matched for age that did not have breast cancer) who had an average ratio of 1.7. This

study, again, confirms that a ratio closer to 2 is significantly safer than a ratio closer to 1.[7]

These studies all show that if you can keep your 2 OH/16 OH ratio (EMI) at 2 or above, you have at least a 30% lower risk of breast cancer than if you allow your ratio (EMI) to drop to 1.5 or below. What happens if your ratio is lower than 1? This study did not specifically discuss the risk to a woman who had a ratio below 1. Most researchers believe that the lower your 2 OH/16 OH ratio (EMI) the higher your risk of breast cancer. In clinical practice, I have seen women with ratios as low as 0.2! These women had a 2 OH/16 OH ratio (EMI) 1/10 the optimal level. Trust me; this is not where YOU want to be.

Why does the 16 OH metabolite significantly increase cancer risk? The 16 OH metabolite maintains strong estrogenic activity, even though it is a metabolite. The stronger the stimulation of your breast tissue, the greater the risk of overstimulation. As we reviewed in Chapter 3, the job of estrogen is to stimulate breast tissue growth. Without estrogen stimulation, your breasts would not have developed in the first place and certainly without estrogen breast health could not be maintained. However, overstimulation causes rapid overproduction of breast cells. If you combine the overproduction of breast cells with lack of control due to DNA (genetic) damage within the nucleus of the cells, the breast cells begin to produce in an out of control manner, leading to breast cancer. (Author's Note: There is some evidence that the 16 OH metabolite may stay bound to the estrogen receptors in your breasts for a long time. This would cause continual stimulation, which as stated above, can lead to overstimulation and overproduction of breast cells.)

The 2 OH metabolite, on the other hand, has low estrogenic activity. This means that when 2 OH binds to the estrogen receptors in your breasts, they stimulate cell reproduction in a more controlled fashion resulting in normal cell multiplication. Therefore, breast cell reproduction does not run wild. If the 2 OH metabolite is bound to an estrogen receptor, 16 OH cannot bind to the same receptor. As you already know, only one estrogen metabolite or estrogen molecule can bind to an estrogen receptor at one time. 2 OH, therefore, helps to protect against the overstimulation that could be caused by the 16 OH metabolite if it could attach to the estrogen receptor.

Why Would Your 2 OH/16 OH Ratio (EMI) be low?

There are multiple reasons.

- Genetics. There are a small percentage of you who have genetic problems with the conversion of estrogen to the 2 OH metabolite. One study done at New York University on African American women found that 8% of the women had an inability or a significantly reduced ability to detoxify estrogen to the 2 OH metabolite, even when exposed to natural substances which improve that conversion. These women are at eight time's greater risk of developing breast cancer than women who do not have this genetic defect.[8] Fortunately, this appears to be a small subset of all women. Why this occurs in up to 8% of African American women is unknown.

- Environmental. There are many environmental factors that cause problems with conversion of estrogen to the 2 OH metabolite: 1) Sluggish liver. If you have reduced amounts of the nutrients necessary to make your P-450 pathway run optimally, you will detoxify estrogen more poorly or convert it to the wrong type of metabolite (i.e. the 16 OH). We will discuss the nutrients that are necessary for proper liver detoxification at length in later chapters. The important point here is that there is a tremendous amount that you can do to improve detoxification of estrogen and shift your detoxification towards the 2 OH pathway. This will cause your 2 OH/16 OH ratio (EMI) to increase, with our goal being 2 or slightly above. If your EMI is below 2, and you are able to improve it to 2 or above, you will reduce your risk of breast cancer by at least 30%. Remember, your estrogen metabolite index (2 OH/16 OH ratio) is the most important predictive factor for breast cancer in post-menopausal women. This makes improving your EMI VITAL if you have a ratio below 2.

How Do You Know What your 2 OH/16 OH Ratio (EMI) Is?

This is the amazing part of our story. Finding out your 2 OH to 16 OH ratio (EMI) is easy and relatively inexpensive. This is usually accomplished via a simple urine test, where we measure the amount of 2 OH and the amount of 16 OH in your urine. In the clinic, I recommend to most women that they obtain a 24-hour urine study which will not only give your EMI (2 OH/16 OH ratio), but will also tell you the levels of your three different estrogens. This will allow you to determine your estrogen quotient (EQ), which is vital in reducing your breast cancer risk. (See Chapters 3 & 4 for a complete discussion of EQ.) If your EMI is not 2 or above, you can make the appropriate changes in your diet and/or add nutritional supplements to increase your ratio and decrease your risk by at least 30%! (If you ask your doctor for a 2 OH to 16 OH ratio, you will more than likely get a very puzzled and/or condescending look. At the end of this book, there is a chapter that talks about the logistics for getting this very easy test completed.)

How Often Should You have Your 2 OH to 16 OH Ratio (EMI) Checked?

Always have your ratio checked before starting supplemental estrogen. In my opinion, every woman should know what her 2 OH/16 OH ratio is. If it is below 2 on your first check, you should recheck it about every 6 months, until it rises to 2 or above. Once you are on a stable program aimed at increasing your EMI (2 OH/16 OH ratio) and your ratio has improved to 2 or above, then you should check it yearly.

Are There Medications that Affect the 2 OH/16 OH (EMI) Ratio?

Certain medications decrease 2 OH and modestly increase 16 OH production. One example is Cimetidine (Tagamet™).[9] If you have recurrent indigestion and require Cimetidine or similar medications frequently, you should work on food allergy avoidance, so that you can reduce your reflux and/or heartburn, and therefore reduce your need for Cimetidine and similar medications. This will help to improve your 2 OH/16 OH ratio. (For a complete discussion of chronic reflux, bowel dysbiosis, and food allergies, see America Exhausted, Breakthrough Treatments of Fatigue and Fibromyalgia; Vitality Press 1998.)

Improving your 2 OH/16 OH ratio. (EMI)

There are several important steps you can take to improve your EMI if it is below 2.

- Improve your diet. Eating more of the nutrients that help you to convert your estrogen to the "good" 2 OH metabolite is an easy first step to take. These nutrients include the cruciferous vegetables which we will discuss at length in the next chapter.

- Improve liver detoxification. Many of you are low in the antioxidants necessary to promote optimal detoxification of estrogen. We will discuss those nutrients in detail in several of the later chapters.

- I3C or DIM. These are nutrients that actually shift your detoxification of estrogen in favor of the 2 OH metabolite. This increases your 2 OH/16 OH ratio (EMI), which is what we have been discussing throughout this chapter. For a complete discussion of I3C and DIM, please see the next chapter.

- Antioxidants. Many antioxidants protect your breast cells from damage, and we will discuss them at length in later chapters.

Summary

There is a tremendous amount you can do to improve your 2 OH/16 OH ratio (EMI). These steps are relatively easy and fairly inexpensive. We will review them in detail throughout the remainder of our time together. The important point to take away from this chapter is you must know what your 2 OH/16 OH ratio is. If it is above 2, terrific! If it is below 2 then you should take steps to improve that ratio to 2 or above. This will reduce your risk of breast cancer by 30% or more. The lower your EMI (2 OH/16 OH ratio), the greater the risk of breast cancer, the more carefully your ratio should be monitored and the more aggressively you should work to improve your ratio. This is something that pre-menopausal women can do to reduce their risk just as easily and effectively as post-menopausal women. If you are in your 20's or 30's, knowing your EMI is vital. Working to make sure it is 2 or above is one of the simple things you can do to significantly reduce your breast cancer risk.

Before we move on to discussing the nutrients that are important for improving your EMI, let's review the third metabolite in figure 5A.

That metabolite is 4 OH (4 Hydroxy-Estrone). 4 OH is a "minor" metabolite. The body converts estrogen predominantly to either the 2 OH or the 16 OH metabolite, with only a small amount being converted to 4 OH. Despite its relatively small amount, 4 OH is a known carcinogen. (In plain English, it is a very bad metabolite.) 4 OH appears to be a free radical generator and may be extremely destructive if you are low in substances that "quench" free radicals. Examples of free radical "quenchers" would be folic acid or the amino acid methionine. Lack of folic acid and/or methionine may contribute to the production of 4 OH. 4 OH causes a special type of destructive free radical named Superoxide. Superoxide radicals are very damaging to DNA. As you already know, the more damage to your DNA, the greater the chances of mutations, which can lead to breast cancer. In one study done on hamsters, 4 OH was shown to be a cancer inducing agent. 4 OH has also been shown to induce breast cancer in human tissue culture.[10] We will discuss folic acid more a little later in its own chapter. It is one of those easy, cheap supplements you can use to significantly reduce your breast cancer risk. Making sure your levels of folic acid stay high, may be one way to prevent excessive 4 OH generation and the Superoxide free radicals that 4 OH produce. Since there are no known adverse side effects to folic acid, at even large doses and it is relatively inexpensive, to me this just seems like a "no brainer".

I promised you that we would review in detail, the nutrients that are available to reduce 16 OH metabolite formation and increase the "good" 2 OH metabolite. Let's move on to the next chapter and discuss I3C and DIM, and review how those breakthrough nutrients can help reduce your risk of breast cancer by 90% or more.

---

[1] Schnieder J, et al., "Abnormal Oxidative Metabolism of Estradiol in Women with Breast Cancer." Proc Nat'l Acad Sci USA (1982); 79:3047-51.

[2] Fishman J, et al., "Increased Estrogen 16-Hydroxylase Activity in Women with Breast and Endometrial Cancer." Journal of Steroid Biochem and Mol Biol (1984); 20: 1077-81.

[3] Sepkovic D W, et al., "Estrogen Metabolite Ratios and Risks Assessment of Hormone Related Cancers: Annals NY Acad Sci (1995); 768:312-16.

[4] Lahita R G, et al., "Increased 16-Hydroxylation of Estradiol in SLE" J Clin Endo Metab (1981);53:174-78

[5] Meilhan EN, et al., "Do Urinary Estrogen Metabolites Predict Breast Cancer?" Guernsey III Cohort follow-up. Today's Journal of Cancer (1998); 78 (9):1250-55.

[6] Luo K W, et al., "Urinary 2/16 Hydroxy Estrone Ratio Correlation with Serum IgF BP3 as a Potential Biomarker of Breast Cancer Risk." Ann Acad Med Singapore (1998); 27 (2):294-99.

[7] Kabat G C, Chang CJ, et al., "Urinary Estrogen Metabolites in Breast Cancer- A Case Controlled Study." Cancer Epidermiological Biomarkers Prev (1997) (7):505-09.

[8] Life Extension: I3C The Tamoxifen Substitute: Cancer Prevention for Thinking People. (Oct 1999):28-34

[9] Michnovicz JJ, Galbraith RA, "Cimetidine Inhibits Catechol Metabolism in Women." Metabolism (1991) (40): 170-74.

[10] Liecht J G, Ricci M J, "4-Hydroxylation of Estrogen as a Marker of Human Mammary Tumors." Proc Nat'l Acad Sci U.S. (1996) (93):3294-96.

6

I3C and DIM: Nature's Secret Weapons

What are I3C and DIM? I3C (Indole-3-Carbinol) is a phyto nutrient that is in cruciferous vegetables. (For a list of cruciferous vegetables see Table 6A.) For years it has been noted that countries that eat more cruciferous vegetables had a lower breast cancer rate than countries who consume less. Until recently, no one has really known why. The reason appears to be that these vegetables contain I3C and the substances that our body makes from I3C, including DIM. When you eat cruciferous vegetables containing I3C, your stomach acid converts the I3C to multiple different compounds. One of those is DIM (Diindolymethane). I3C and/or DIM can reduce your risk of breast cancer in three ways.

Table 6A cruciferous vegetables (Brassica)

• Cabbage	• Brussel sprouts
• Broccoli	• Bok choy
• Cauliflower	• Collards
• Kale	• Turnips
• Watercress	• Rutabaga

1) I3C and DIM improve the way you metabolize estrogen. In the last chapter we discussed how estrogen is converted to two predominant metabolites, 2 OH and 16 OH. You learned that if you convert your

estrogen primarily to the 16 OH metabolite, your risk of breast cancer INCREASES. You also learned that if you convert more of your estrogen to the 2 OH metabolite, your risk DECREASES. You learned how important your 2 OH/16 OH ratio (estrogen metabolic index or EMI) is to cancer prevention. We discussed that if your 2 OH/16 OH ratio was low, there are several natural steps you can take to improve it. I3C and DIM are two natural substances that improve your 2 OH/16 OH ratio. How? I3C/DIM up regulates the conversion of estrogen to the 2 OH metabolite. It does this by increasing the enzyme that converts Estradiol or Estrone to 2 OH. (That enzyme is named 2 alpha hydroxylase.) When you eat vegetables that contain I3C that I3C is converted in your stomach to DIM and the DIM shifts your conversion towards the "good" 2 OH metabolite and away from the "bad" 16 OH metabolite. This, by definition, improves your 2 OH/16 OH ratio (EMI). See figure 6B. Since I3C/DIM helps to convert your estrogen towards the "good" 2 OH metabolite, there is less estrogen available to be converted to the 16 OH "bad" metabolite. Studies have shown that I3C begins to improve 2 hydroxylation, (this conversion to the 2 OH metabolite) in as little as five days of use.[1] The improvement lasted as long as the I3C was taken and no major side effects were noted. [1] A study done on 60 women, with 20 of them getting 400 mg I3C a day, the other 40 getting either placebo or cellulose (fiber), showed the 2 OH/16 OH ratio increased for the group on I3C and stayed up for the full three months of the study, without apparent harmful side effects. In another study published in the Journal of the National Cancer Institute, 10 women were given 400 mg I3C for two months. I3C increased their urinary excretion of 2 OH, (This means 2 OH levels went up, so more was excreted in the urine) and the Estrone (E1) +

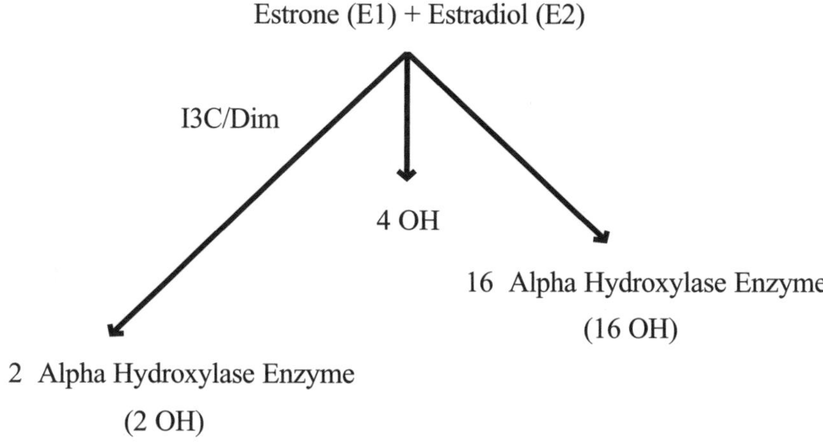

Figure 6B

Estradiol (E2) urine levels of more harmful estrogen and 16 OH metabolites went DOWN![2] These harmful estrogens included Estradiol, Estrone and the 16 OH metabolite. It should be noted that the reduction in 16 OH will improve your EMI, and the reduction of Estradiol and Estrone will improve your estrogen quotient (EQ). Both of these changes powerfully reduce your risk of breast cancer.

2.) I3C/DIM improves the function of tumor suppressor genes. I3C and DIM appear to work on both estrogen receptor positive (ER positive), breast cancer cells and estrogen receptor negative (ER negative). (Author's Note: ER positive breast cancers require estrogen to allow them to grow. ER negative breast cancers do not require the presence of estrogen to grow, and therefore respond much more poorly to estrogen receptor modulating agents, such as Tamoxifen and/or Raloxifene.) I3C works on ER negative breast cancer, by being able to up regulate your cancer suppressor genes BRCA-1 and P21. Remember from Chapter one that BRCA-1 slows breast cell reproduction and is one of the genes responsible for keeping cell reproduction under control.[3,4] The absolutely fascinating results of these studies showed that I3C slowed the growth of ER negative cancer cells by 50%. It did this by improving the function of BRCA-1 and P21.[11] (Author's Note: We did not discuss P21 in our genetics chapter, but it is an important tumor suppressor gene, along with BRCA-1 and BRCA-2.) You will be hearing a lot about BRCA-1, especially since a test is now available to identify women with inherited BRCA-1 or BRCA-2 mutations. (See Chapter 1) What no physician tells you is that breast cancer tumor suppressor genes can actually be up regulated both by foods and/or supplements. You can bet that if a pharmaceutical company held a patent on I3C/DIM, every other television commercial would "inform you" on the benefits of taking that medicine. Since I3C/DIM are natural substances and cannot be patented, no one is "bothering" to inform you. Important Point: I will repeat, research shows that the I3C in vegetables or I3C/DIM by supplement can improve how your tumor suppressor genes, BRCA-1 and P21 function, therefore, significantly reducing your risk of breast cancer. I3C improved BRCA-1 in both estrogen receptor positive (MCF-7) and estrogen receptor negative (MDA-MB-468) breast cancer cells.[4] If this one fact was not good enough reason to eat the cruciferous vegetables, we also know from research that I3C up regulates the effects of the invasion suppressor complex named E-cadherin. If the E-cadherin complex is not functioning properly, it allows breast cancer to invade surrounding normal tissue. As the study states, "Restoration of E-cadherin is able to dramatically suppressive invasive phenotypes".[4] (Author's Interpretation: If you restore your E-cadherin complex, you dramatically reduce or suppress those breast cancers which invade more aggressively. Those tumors that invade most aggressively are the most dangerous and the most likely to kill you. The importance of restoration of E-cadherin cannot be overemphasized.) So the studies have shown I3C has been found to up regulate tumor suppressor genes BRCA-1 and P21 AND improve the function of tumor invasion suppressor substances, such as the E-cadherin complex.

3.) I3C/DIM blocks cancer causing chemicals from attaching to the estrogen receptors in your breasts. I3C/DIM bind to the aryl hydrocarbon receptor in your breast cells. (Aryl hydrocarbon receptor is also called the "Ah" receptor.) The "Ah" receptor stimulates cell growth. Chemicals such as dioxin, when attached to the "Ah" receptor, cause breast cells to reproduce wildly, eventually resulting in a tumor. [11] (Author's Note: We will discuss dioxin at length in the Chemical Carcinogen's Chapter. In that chapter you will see that dioxin is nearly everywhere, including our food. So most of you have dioxin in you now and consume small amounts of dioxin daily.)

If I3C is attached to the "Ah" receptor, dioxin cannot bind. If dioxin cannot bind, it cannot overstimulate breast cells; therefore, breast cell reproduction stays at a normal level. Dioxin appears to activate cancer growth genes and suppress tumor suppressor genes. In one study I3C reduced chemically caused breast cancer in rodents by 70-90%.[11] Another study, done at Texas A & M University showed that I3C reduced the cancer promotion effects of dioxin on breast cells by 90%.[5] Unfortunately, I3C does not stay bound to the "Ah" receptor for long periods of time. Therefore, one should take small amounts of I3C/DIM on a regular basis to maintain its competitive inhibition of dioxin and related organochlorines. (Author's Note: Studies have shown that once dioxin binds to your estrogen receptor it may be irreversible, causing continued long-term stimulation of your breast tissue. This may be the reason it causes your breast cell reproduction to run wild eventually causing a tumor.)

DIM (Diindolymethane).

We have been using I3C and DIM interchangeably throughout the course of this chapter. Let's review briefly what DIM is and the differences between I3C and DIM. DIM is one of the active metabolites of I3C. I3C does not appear to have any direct effect in the body. When you eat vegetables that contain I3C, it requires stomach acid to convert the I3C to its metabolites. The amount of stomach acid determines what metabolites you make. If your stomach acid is low, you have more difficulty utilizing I3C, and your conversion of I3C to DIM is less efficient. Despite what the commercials are constantly telling you, millions of you have low stomach acid, especially if you are over the age of 40. One of the great ironies of life is that low stomach acid can actually create many of the same symptoms that "high" stomach acid creates: poor digestion, indigestion, bloating and gas. Lack of proper stomach acid causes poor absorption of many nutrients, including I3C. Millions of you are on acid suppression medications for chronic acid reflux disease. These medications reduce the absorption of I3C by lowering stomach acid. (Author's Note: Unfortunately, physicians prescribe these acid suppressive medications routinely instead of looking for the real cause of the chronic reflux, which in many cases is caused by chronic food allergies, bacterial infections such as h- pylori, yeast infections such as candida, and/or lack of digestive enzymes.) If you are on an acid suppressive medication, you will have difficulty converting I3C to DIM, therefore, a DIM supplement may be required. Even under conditions of normal stomach pH, only about 10% of I3C is converted to DIM.[6] As we briefly reviewed, I3C is not only converted to DIM, but multiple other phyto chemicals, including ICZ, IAN, CTR, ASG and LTR. The effects of these phyto chemical metabolites are not well known at this time. There is considerable controversy concerning the question, "Will these metabolites, in high doses, cause side effects?" For example, ICZ (indolocarbazole) is estrogenic and has been shown to promote enzymes which increase the 4 OH metabolites of estrogen. [12] We reviewed in the last chapter that 4 OH has been associated with increasing the risk of breast cancer and/or uterine tumors. [7] With this in mind, increasing levels of ICZ may not be such a great idea. Studies have shown that DIM (Diindolymethane) improves the production of the "good" 2 OH metabolite through increasing the activity of 2 alpha hydroxylase (the enzymes that converts estrogen to 2 OH).[8] Research has shown that DIM blocks the "Ah" receptor as effectively as I3C. DIM improves your EMI (2 OH/16 OH ratio) at a lower dose than I3C and with less possible side effects. Most research points to DIM as being the most important breakdown product of I3C. [10,] DIM up regulates the activity of your liver enzymes without elevating the quantity. It does not appear to affect the enzymes, which increase the metabolism of various drugs. Therefore, it should not interfere with medications as much as I3C.[10,12] It is up to 10 times more active than I3C, so smaller amounts need to be taken if a supplement is used.[12] For the millions of people with low stomach acid either through age related decline or reduction via acid suppression medication, DIM is the supplement of choice, since it does not require normal stomach acid for absorption, and as we have already reviewed, I3C is impacted rather significantly by reduced stomach acid. (Hypochlorhydria)

I3C versus DIM—The Controversy.

Recently a controversy has developed as to which is the superior supplement I3C or DIM? The group that supports I3C believes that several of the breakdown products of I3C may be important for breast cancer prevention. They point out that when you take a DIM supplement, you only get DIM and that if other breakdown products are important you would miss out on those benefits. The other group, including the company that owns the patent on absorbable DIM, counters with studies that show certain metabolites of I3C like ICZ and ascorbigen (ASB) may increase the production of the 4 OH metabolite, which increases the risk of breast cancer. [9] Furthermore, they feel that since DIM appears to be responsible for many, if not all, of the positive effects of I3C on estrogen detoxification, and that DIM appears safer and it should be the supplement of choice. This becomes a controversy only if you decide to use supplemental I3C or DIM to improve your 2 OH/16 OH ratio. It should be noted the cruciferous vegetables contain I3C, which is then converted in your stomach to DIM, along with multiple other metabolites, and since eating cruciferous vegetables is the most natural treatment, this is where you should start. I recognize, however, many of you will not eat cruciferous vegetables and will want the ease and/or convenience of taking a supplement. In addition, some of you may have a very low EMI and may not be able to eat enough of the cruciferous vegetables to improve your ratio to our target, which is 2 or above. For you, supplementation with I3C or DIM would be reasonable. At this time, supplementation with DIM appears to be the safer of the two choices. In addition it has the following positive points:

1. It improves 2 OH, and therefore raises your EMI (2 Oh/16 OH ratio).

2. Smaller doses are required to obtain an effect, therefore the possibility of side effects are reduced.

3. DIM has the ability to block the "Ah" receptor in your breasts, and therefore protect your breasts from the dangerous/toxic effects of chemicals like dioxin.

4. It is unclear from studies if DIM improves BRCA-1 or P21 function, but since it is the major active metabolite of I3C, it would stand to reason that it does. Further studies on this one issue need to be conducted.

5. H. Leon Bradlow, PhD of the Strang Cancer Research Center in New York, one of the pioneer researchers on the effects of I3C on estrogen metabolism, has come out publicly in favor of DIM as opposed to I3C as a supplement. Although much of Dr. Bradlow's original research was done with I3C, after reviewing new research, he feels that DIM is the safer form of supplement.

Summary

Step One: Know what your EMI (2 OH/16 OH ratio) is.

Step Two: If it is below 2, add as many of the cruciferous vegetables to your diet as possible.

Step Three: If your ratio does not improve to 2 or more and you are unable and/or unwilling to eat cruciferous vegetables, then add low doses of bioavailable DIM beginning at 75 mg once daily. Recheck your EMI (2 OH/16 OH ratio) in 6 months.

Step Four: If upon recheck your EMI it is still below 2, increase your DIM to 150 mg per day and recheck your ratio in 6 months.

Step Five: If you are a plus-sized woman and your 2 OH/16 OH ratio (EMI) is still below 2 after taking the 150 mg of DIM for six months, then increase up to 300 mg per day. Recheck your EMI in 6 months.

Caution: These are general guidelines. Never begin a supplement program without the approval of your medical professional.

Possible Side Effects.

1. If you get your I3C through cruciferous vegetables, there is very little risk of side effects, except perhaps excessive gas.

2. DIM (absorbable Diindolymethane): NEVER use DIM or I3C if you are pregnant or breast feeding. Although there are no studies showing that they are toxic, there also are no human studies on the safety of DIM/I3C during pregnancy and/or breast feeding. Therefore, avoid it.

3. CAUTION with using DIM/I3C and birth control pills (PCPs/oral contraceptives). No formal studies of DIM/I3C and birth control pills have been completed. If you wish to use DIM/I3C, then add additional birth control methods. Example: barrier plus condoms.

4. Always take DIM/I3C with food.

5. Headaches. Occasional headaches have been noted with DIM. If this happens, reduce your dose until the headache subsides, then increase the dose more slowly.

6. Nausea. If this occurs, it is usually relieved by taking DIM with food.

7. Diarrhea. This is rare, but if it happens, reduce your dose.

8. Urine color. Urine color may change to amber. This is harmless but should reduce with increasing your fluid intake. [12]

Conclusion

You now know that a 2 OH/16 OH ratio (EMI) less than 2 significantly INCREASES your risk of breast cancer. If your ratio is below 2, nature has given you a secret weapon that will allow you to raise your EMI and REDUCE your breast cancer risk. That weapon is named I3C/DIM. If your EMI is low, start eating your cruciferous vegetables! If after six months it is still low, or if you are unwilling and/or unable to eat cruciferous vegetables, the addition of a low dose DIM/I3C, in my opinion, would seem prudent. Combine these dietary changes with the remainder of the program that we will discuss, including increasing your tocotrienols, lowering hydrogenated fat, increasing omega 3 fatty acids, increasing your B-12/folic acid and adding curcumin to your diet. We will review each one of these recommendations in full detail in later chapters. If you make these easy changes, you are well on your way to reducing your risk of breast cancer by 90% OR MORE!

---

[1] Bradlow H et al., "I3C, A Novel Approach to Breast Cancer Prevention" Ann NY Acad Sci (1995); 76:180-200.

[2] Michnovicz JJ et al., "Changes in Levels of Urinary Estrogen Metabolites After I3C Treatment in Humans" Journal National Cancer Institute, Volume 89 No 10 (21 May 1997)

[3] Cover C et al.,

[4] Meng Q et al., "Suppression of Breast Cancer Invasion and Migration by I3C" J Mol Med (2000); 78:155-65.

[5] Chen I, Safe S, Bjeldanes L: "Indole 3- Carbinol and Diindolymethane as Aryl Hydrocarbon (Ah) Receptor Agonists and Antagonists in T47D Human Breast Cancer Cells" Biochemical Pharmacology, Vol 51:1069-76 (1996)

[6] DeKruif CA et al., "Structure Elucidation of Acid Reaction Products of I3C: Detection in Vivo and Enzyme Induction in Vitro" Chem Biol Interact (1991); 80 (3):303-15.

[7] Hayes CL, Spink DC, Spink BC et al., "17-beta Estradiol Hydroxylation Catalyzed by Human Cytocrome P450 1B1" Pro Nat'l Acad Sci USA (1996) (3 Sept 93) (18):7996-81.

[8] Jellinck PH et al., "Ah Receptor Binding Properties of Indole Carbinols and Induction of Hepatic Estradiol Hydroxylation" Biochem Pharmaceutical (1993); 45:1129-36.

[9] Sepkovic DW et al., "Catechol Estrogen Production in Rat Microsomes After Treatment with I3C, Ascorbigen or Beta-Naphtha flavone Steroids" (1994 May); 59 (5):318-23.

10 Zeligs MA, "Safer Estrogen with Phyto nutrition" Townsend Letter for Doctors & Patients (April 1999)
11 "I3C The Tamoxifen Substitute Cancer Prevention for Thinking People" Life Extension (Oct 1999):28-34.
12 Zeligs MA "DIM and I3C: The Real Facts on Safety" Vol. 1,2 :1-14

7

Phytoestrogens and Protection From Breast Cancer

What are phytoestrogens, and how do they help protect you from breast cancer? The word phytoestrogen is actually a misnomer, since plants do not make estrogen, only animals produce true estrogen. The term phytoestrogen refers to nutrients in certain plants whose chemical structure allows them to bind with your estrogen receptors. These substances, in many cases, have chemical structures that are similar to 17 beta-Estradiol. (See figure 7A.)

These phytoestrogens occur in nature as two major classes: Isoflavones and lignans. Isoflavones are found predominantly in the legume family, this includes soy. Lignans are found in whole grains, legumes, vegetables and seeds, especially flaxseed.

The medical literature shows that women who have higher levels of phytoestrogens in their urine have a significantly reduced risk of breast cancer. One study published in the British Medical Journal showed that there was a fourfold risk reduction for women in the highest 25% of excretion of the phytoestrogen Equol vs the women in the lowest 25% of excretion. [1] In other words, those women who were in the highest 25% of Equol excretion had a four times lower risk of breast cancer than the 25% who had the lowest levels. This same study showed that the 25% of women who excreted the most of the phytoestrogen Enterolactone were at 1/3 the risk of breast cancer as the 25% of women who excreted the least. One-third the risk! According

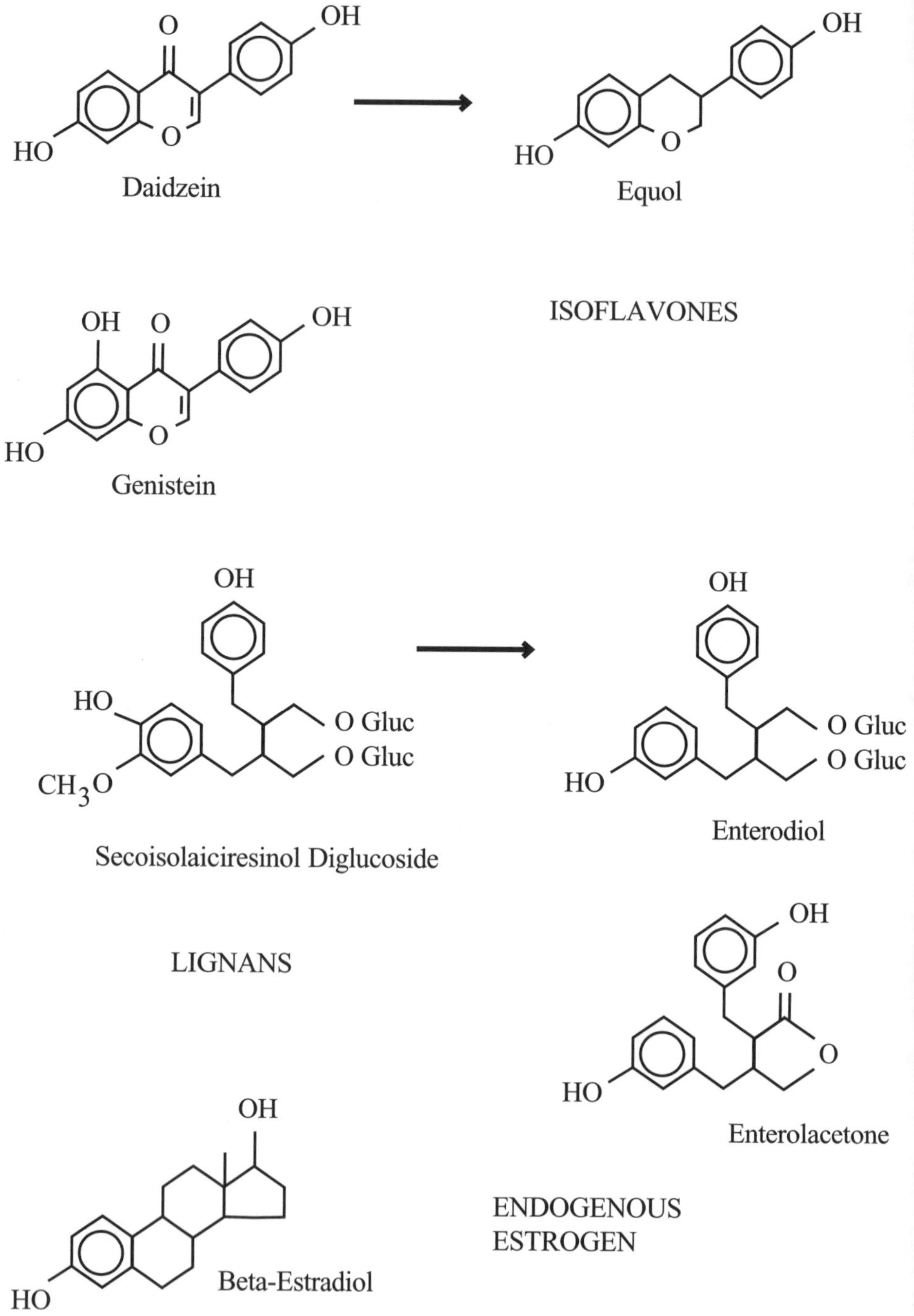

Daidzein

Equol

Genistein

ISOFLAVONES

Secoisolaiciresinol Diglucoside

Enterodiol

LIGNANS

Enterolacetone

Beta-Estradiol

ENDOGENOUS ESTROGEN

Figure 7A

to the study, these results were true for both pre-menopausal and post-menopausal women.[1]

Two other studies also showed that phytoestrogen excretion was lower in women with breast cancer than in the control groups (women without breast cancer, approximately the same age).[2,3] A fascinating article appeared in a recent edition of the Journal Carcinogenesis, September 2002. Researchers at USC found that Asian-American women who reported eating soy weekly, when they were adolescents and now as adults, had a 47% reduction in breast cancer risk compared to those who ate low levels of soy. For the women who ate high levels of soy as adolescents, but now eat low levels as an adult, the risk was still 23% lower. The greatest percentage of risk reduction was found in those women who ate the highest amount of soy.[4] (This study was done via interview of 501 Asian-American women with breast cancer and 594 healthy Asian-American women.)

Study 5.

A study published in the Journal of Cancer, Epidemiology, Biomarkers and Prevention, September 2002, showed that post-menopausal women in Singapore who ate soy based foods regularly as part of their diet, had lower levels of Estrone vs those women who did not eat soy. (Author's Note: Remember, we have discussed Estrone is a strong estrogen that lowers your estrogen quotient and increases your risk of breast cancer.) Those women in the top 25% of soy consumption had Estrone levels 15% lower than the other 75% of the women in the study.[5] Are you starting to get the impression that it would be to your benefit to be in the top 25% of women in soy consumption? One study showing you can reduce your risk by four times, another showing a 47% reduction in risk, and two others showing phytoestrogen excretion was lowest in women with breast cancer.

Why do women who consume high levels of phytoestrogens have lower breast cancer risks?

There are several possible mechanisms:

- Phytoestrogens bind estrogen receptors and exert a weak estrogen-like activity. When phytonutrients are bound to the estrogen receptors, they reduce the amount of strong estrogens that can attach. This blocks Estradiol, Estrone and the 16 OH metabolite from binding and therefore overstimulating your breast tissue. We have already discussed that Estradiol, Estrone and 16 OH are strong stimulators of cell reproduction. You know that overstimulation by these strong estrogens can cause cellular reproduction to go out of control, (if there is DNA damage) eventually resulting in a tumor. If you keep many of the estrogen receptors occupied by a weak estrogenic substance, you significantly reduce the possibility of overstimulation from the strong estrogens and estrogen metabolites. This reduces your cancer risk. For years researchers have wondered why Japanese women have a significantly lower risk of breast cancer compared with American women. Yet, when Oriental women adopt a Western diet, their incidence of breast cancer elevates to the Western level within two generations. [6] (Author's Note: Breast cancer rates have historically been 4-7 times higher in the United States than in China or Japan. This will probably change, as we send the children of China and Japan burgers and fries. As that generation drifts away from the traditional diet one would expect their level of breast cancer to start going up exponentially.)

Studies have shown that the reduction in breast cancer of Oriental women is not genetic since those women studied who moved to the United States changed their diet, but did not significantly alter their gene pool. In addition, two generations is a very short time to alter your gene pool, therefore, it is doubtful that the elevation of breast cancer incidence of Oriental women who adopt a Western diet is secondary to genetic causes. Almost certainly the increase in risk is secondary to diet.

Many studies have shown that Oriental women consume large amounts of the foods that contain phytoestrogens, particularly soy products like tofu, soy sprouts, tempeh, bean paste and miso. Oriental women have levels of phytoestrogens anywhere from 100 to 1000 times that typical of a Western woman.[7] Many Asian women consume 20-80 mg a day of the phytoestrogen Genistein. The estimated amount a woman in the United States consumes is approximately 1-3 mg daily.[8]

- Phytoestrogens may alter the 2 OH/16 OH ratio (EMI). A study published in 1998 showed that post-menopausal women who had their diet supplemented with soy powder had increased levels of the 2 OH metabolite, and a decrease in 16 OH, 4 OH, and Estradiol. The study suggested that "soy Isoflavones may exert a cancer preventative affect by altering metabolism away from the genotoxic metabolites and toward weaker metabolites". 12

- Soy phytoestrogens lower blood levels of the more dangerous estrogens. Earlier we reviewed the new study published in Cancer Epidemiology, Biomarkers and Prevention, showing that eating soy foods on a regular basis lowered the serum levels of the strong estrogen Estrone. High levels of Estrone have been associated with an increased risk of breast cancer. We have just discussed a study showing that soy protein appears to increase your 2 OH and decrease 16 OH, 4 OH and Estradiol.

Summary

Review of the medical literature seems clear that phytoestrogens are important for reducing your risk of breast cancer. They appear to do so by three important mechanisms.

1. They bind to the estrogen receptors and do not allow the stronger, more stimulatory, estrogens or estrogen metabolites to attach.

2. They alter your 2 OH to 16 OH ratio (EMI), causing an elevation of 2 OH and a reduction of 16 OH, therefore improving your EMI.

3. They appear to lower the blood levels of the more dangerous estrogens Estrone and Estradiol.

We have known for decades that Oriental women have a significantly lower breast cancer incidence, as compared with those women who eat a Western diet. We now, through medical studies, appear to know the reason why. We have evidence from the real world and evidence from the research world on why increasing your levels of phytoestrogens seems logical and beneficial. The majority of women that I have seen in the clinic really have no problem understanding and accepting the fact that they should increase their phytonutrient intake. The problems arise when they try to do this on a day to day basis in the real world. In the Orient, it is much easier, since many of their foods are soy based. Soy has become part of their culture. In the Western diet, this is quite the opposite. Let's review some easy ways to increase your phytoestrogen intake.

<u>Soy</u>

The first step that should always be taken is to increase the soy foods in your diet. The easiest way to get soy protein is to mix soy powder with soy milk once daily in the blender. I have recommended this to women for years, since it is a cheap and easy way to get a large amount of soy Isoflavones in your diet with very little fuss. Most women will mix this up in the morning and sip it with breakfast or on their way to work. They find it is very easy and convenient. Recently, however, some scientists have started to question the value of using non-fermented soy products. They note that the soy intake of Oriental women consists overwhelmingly of foods that are fermented. Example: miso, tempeh and tofu. (Tofu is prepared in a slightly different manner that still allows the soy protein to be broken down.) One long-time researcher/doctor looked back into ancient Chinese writings and found that soy beans were not added to the Chinese diet until a process was discovered to remove toxins. Once this fermentation process was discovered, soy became a staple of the Chinese diet.[13] The question is why did the ancient Chinese not eat non-fermented soy foods? The answer may be that along with phytonutrients, soy also contains other substances that may interfere with health. These substances include phytic acid, enzyme inhibitors and possibly substances that interfere with thyroid function. Phytic acid has been reported to bind several minerals, including zinc, copper, iron, magnesium and calcium. Therefore, consumption of large amounts of phytic acid may place a drain on the mineral levels in your body. Fermentation breaks down much of the phytic acid. Soaking in water also reduces the phytic acid content of soy. [13]

Goitrogens

It has been reported that unfermented soy contains substances that interfere with thyroid function. These substances are named goitrogens. Animals fed unfermented soy have been known to have an increased risk of goiter. [13] Many American women are low in thyroid function and do not know it. Many have mild or not so mild thyroid inflammation named thyroiditis. Once again, fermentation appears to break down these goitrogens and allow soy to be consumed without harmful effects on the thyroid. [11] It should be noted, that no large scale studies have been conducted to find out if eating raw soy in large amounts is harmful or not. It is very interesting that a society that loves soy and has it integrated so finely in their diet, does not eat very much in the way of raw soy. One of my theories has always been, when the studies are in question or unclear, one should proceed with what has worked. We know that Oriental women have a significantly lower risk of breast cancer than Western women. We also know that Oriental women eat large amounts of fermented soy products, and therefore consume vastly more Isoflavones than women on a Western diet. Furthermore, studies have shown these Isoflavones improve your EMI, improve your EQ, and bind the estrogen receptors in your breasts not allowing the stronger estrogens to attach. Until the question about fermented vs unfermented soy is answered, I recommend adding fermented soy products to your diet, such as tofu, mizo and tempah. Our goal would be to add roughly 20 mg of genistein per day to your overall diet. For a list of foods that contain genistein see Figure 7B. There are many books where you can find delicious, easy recipes that will help you incorporate more soy foods into your diet and your daughter's diet. Remember the study that showed that women who started phytoestrogen foods at a younger age had a significantly reduced level of breast cancer as opposed to those women who had just eaten soy foods as adults. I understand this may take some work. Probably the first food a young woman would accept and eat would be tofu, used in appropriate recipes.

Food		Genistein *
Tofu	100 grams	15 mg
Tempeh	50 grams	17 mg
Bean Curd	100 grams	25 mg
Bean Paste	100 grams	25 mg
Roasted Soybeans	20 grams	18 mg

Ref 14 *Approximate Levels

Figure 7B

Flaxseed

Flax is a major source of the phytoestrogen lignan. (See Figure 7A.) The normal level of lignans for a woman on a Western diet is: Enterolactone 3.2 umol per day and Enterodiol 1.3 umol per day. Look what happens to those levels when you take 10 grams of flaxseed powder daily: Eterolactone 27.8 umol per day, Enterodiol 19.5 umol per day. [6] (These were urinary measurements). Ten grams of flaxseed a day raised both of the phytoestrogen levels by over 10 times. Studies of urinary lignans in post-menopausal women showed that lignan levels were significantly lower in the women with breast cancer vs normal women. [2,3]

The mechanisms for how flaxseed can reduce your risk of breast cancer are similar to soy. The phytoestrogens in flax, namely, Enterolactone and Enterodiol bind to estrogen receptors in your breasts and exert very weak estrogenic activity. This estrogenic activity is one reason why post-menopausal women have found soy and flax helpful in controlling menopausal symptoms. (We will discuss this in detail later in this chapter.) As we reviewed with soy, if a weak phytoestrogenic substance is bound to the estrogen receptors, the stronger estrogens and estrogen metabolites cannot bind. This lowers breast cell stimulation and keeps breast tissue reproduction at more normal levels. It is unclear at this time if flax phytoestrogens also improves your EMI. The author was not able to find any studies on flax phytoestrogens and the EMI.

Flaxseed can be bought at any health food store and ground into a powder, using an electric coffee grinder or food processor. This powder can be added to just about anything; soups, salads, breads, muffins, meat loaf or eaten by itself as a warm cereal in winter. This is an extremely cheap, easy and good tasting way to get your phytoestrogens. In one study conducted at a major university on the East Coast, that is ongoing as we speak, they are using flax muffins containing 10 grams of flax powder, and women eat one muffin a day.

Osteoporosis and Phytoestrogens.

It is becoming clear that phytoestrogens can play a part in prevention of osteoporosis. A study published in The American Journal of Clinical Nutrition showed that high levels of soy Isoflavones protected against spinal bone loss. [7] This study was done on 66 post-menopausal women who had high cholesterol. Significant increases in bone mineral content and density occurred in the group that was given 40 grams of isolated soy protein per day, which contained 2.25 mg of Isoflavones per gram of protein. In addition, this study also showed that Isoflavones from soy decreased the risk factors that cause heart disease.

For decades researchers/doctors have struggled to explain a paradox (or what appeared to be a paradox). Oriental women would seem to be perfect candidates for osteoporosis. They are fair-skinned, usually small-boned, and live in a northern climate. Yet the risk of osteoporosis in Japan is significantly lower than the risk in the United States, Canada or Northern Europe. One reason for this may be that soy Isoflavones help reduce bone loss. Studies done in the U.S. so far have been conflicting, with some studies showing improvement in bone density, others showing none. Yet there are some studies, like the one I just quoted, that shows a clear association between higher Isoflavone levels and prevention of spinal bone loss. It should be noted that Oriental women have higher levels of phytoestrogens from childhood. This long level of exposure may help protect them from bone loss, beginning at age 30. Remember, you do not just lose bone starting at menopause. The pace of bone loss increases dramatically after menopause, but most women begin to lose bone after age 30. There could be other factors involved in this paradox. Oriental women consume more fish, and therefore more vitamin D. They obtain their calcium through different foods than Western women. There could be differences in the quality of calcium or vitamin D that Oriental women are getting in their diet, therefore causing less bone loss. Phytoestrogens do not reduce bone loss as well as supplemental estrogen, but as we have already discussed, the strong estrogens raise your breast cancer risk. We should note that it appears to be more beneficial to have moderate amounts of phytoestrogens over longer periods of time vs high amounts of phytoestrogens for short periods of time. Certainly in the United States, we have the philosophy that more is better and quicker is best. Yet when we look at societies with low breast cancer levels and low osteoporosis rates, it would seem reasonable that a moderate amount of phytoestrogens and/or cruciferous vegetables taken over longer periods of time are more productive than higher amounts used for shorter periods. This is the reason why I want you to find good tasting recipes for cruciferous vegetables, soy, and flax. You need to make these a part of your everyday diet for life. The best way to do this is to find recipes that you enjoy. Obviously, if you hate what you are eating, you will not do it for long. Experiment and find those recipes you enjoy and use them.

Phytoestrogens and Postmenopausal Symptom Improvement.

Many women have noted improvement in hot flashes, night sweats, and sleep disturbances with phytoestrogen supplementation. In the next chapter, we will discuss a particular supplement named Black Cohosh. Many of my patients have used soy and flax to control postmenopausal symptoms. By doing so, they receive many benefits.

1. They reduce their symptoms, since the soy/flax Isoflavones act as very weak estrogenic substances. By fitting into estrogen receptors, they mimic the effect of estrogen, but very weakly.

2. They reduce the risk of breast cancer through soy/flax's ability to improve the EQ, improve the EMI and bind the estrogen receptors.

3. They probably reduce the rate of spinal bone loss.

4. They get a great tasting source of high-quality protein. Soy seems to work better for women in perimenopause or early menopause. Yet, I have seen women who are in the middle of menopause have their symptoms controlled very nicely.

It is interesting that some Oriental cultures do not have a word for menopause. This could be due to the fact that Oriental women are consuming so much soy Isoflavones that the symptoms of menopause are relatively benign. If you can control your menopausal symptoms with soy and/or other phytoestrogens, this would be the safest treatment available. Even though phytoestrogens have some very mild estrogenic activity, no studies have shown any association between phytoestrogens and increased risk of breast cancer. Every study this author has found has shown a correlation between phytoestrogens and decreased risk. A note for women who have had breast cancer: The majority of women who have had breast cancer, particularly if it is estrogen receptor positive, have been told not to use phytoestrogen nutrients and/or supplements, for fear that mild estrogenic stimulation would cause a return of the breast cancer. This is one of those difficult questions for which there is no "right" answer for everyone. If you are menopausal and have had breast cancer, but you are miserable, cannot sleep, cannot think, sexual function is poor with hot flashes and night sweats increasing the phytoestrogen foods in your diet could be a good first step. Clinically, I have worked with many women on this very complex issue. Their quality of life is poor. They are scared to death of getting breast cancer again, and they did not tolerate or did not want to take the selected estrogen receptor modulators (SERMS; Example Tamoxifen and/or Raloxifene). I have reviewed the pros and cons of all of the therapies we have discussed in this book with those women. Of course, the final decision must be theirs, as they must accept the responsibility for their actions and their health. Many women have wished to try a middle-of-the-road approach. They have found their quality of life to be unacceptable without any estrogen modulation. Yet, they are scared to death to take an estrogen supplement, even Estriol. Many of them have chosen to increase the phytoestrogens in their diet to see if it will make the symptoms more manageable, while still maintaining minimal estrogenic stimulation to their breasts. To my knowledge, no clear-cut study has been completed showing phytoestrogen either reducing or increasing the risk of <u>recurrent</u> breast cancer. This is a study that desperately needs to be done. Unfortunately, there is very little incentive for the pharmaceutical industry or our government to proceed with that study. I suppose we will have to do it. In any case, as I said before, never proceed with any supplementation without the expressed consent of your physician.* If you have had breast cancer, proceeding with high-dosed soy protein supplementation is <u>not</u> the first step. Changes in your diet would be the first step to see if that will make your symptoms more manageable.

<u>Summary</u>

Studies have shown:

1. Phytoestrogens genistein, daidzein, equol, enterolactone, and enterodiol have been associated with <u>reduction</u> in the risk of breast cancer.

2. Asian populations who consume 100 to 1000 times the level of phytoestrogens of Western women, have <u>4-7 times</u> lower risk of breast cancer. In studies, those Oriental women who were the highest 25% in phytoestrogen consumption had a <u>4 times</u> lower risk than those Oriental women in the lowest 25%. Remember, even the Oriental women in the lowest group have a 4-7 times lower risk of breast cancer than YOU.

3. Soy consumption is an excellent way to increase the phytoestrogens genistein, diadzein, and equol. Due to possible questions concerning side effects from raw or unfermented soy products, I recommend using the fermented soy products tofu, mizo and tempah as part of a change in your everyday diet. Your goal should be, roughly, 20-30 mg of genistein per day, which is equal to roughly 25-50 grams of soy protein per day.

4. Ground flaxseed is an excellent source of the lignans enterodiol and enterolactone. Your goal should be to get 10-25 grams of flaxseed per day via various wholesome, great-tasting foods. At minimum, eat one flax muffin containing 10 grams of ground flaxseed daily or several times per week.

*Use a physician knowledgeable of phytoestrogens and their use in menopause.

5. Even if you cannot eat the recommended amount of soy and/or flax per day, do it as many times per week as possible. Consuming some soy and/or flax over the course of many months should confer some protective effect and reduce your risk of breast cancer. I want to emphasize it is better to eat moderate amounts of soy and/or flax several times a week for years than to eat larger amounts and then burn out and quit. There are many other health benefits associated with phyto nutrient consumption, which we will not review in this book. These include reduction of several other types of cancer and as I mentioned earlier, reduction in risk of heart disease.

Final Note

For those of you who wish, urinary evaluations of phytoestrogens are available as part of the 24-hour urine estrogen evaluation we previously mentioned. If you are interested in this or further information, please see the product resource chapter at the end of this book.

---

[1] Ingram D, et al., "Case Controlled Study of Phytoestrogens and Breast Cancer" Lancet, Vol. 350 (4 Oct 1997):990-94.

[2] Adlercreutzh H et al., "Excretion of the Lignans, Enterolactone and Enterodiol and of Equol in Omnivorous and Vegetarian Postmenopausal Women and in Women with Breast Cancer" Lancet (11 Dec. 1982):1295-98.

[3] Ziegler et al., "Migration Patterns and Breast Cancer Risk in Asian American Women" Journal of National Cancer Institute, Vol. 85 (22) (17 Nov. 1993)

[4] Adlercreutz H "Dietary Phytoestrogens and the Menopause in Japan" Lancet, Vol. 339 (16 May 1992)

[5] Barnes S et al., "Rationale for the use of Genistein Containing Soy Matrices in Chemoprevention Trials for Breast and Prostate Cancer" Journal of Cell Biochem (1995); 22:181-87.

[6] Cassidy A Binghams et al., "Biological Effects of Isoflavones in Young Women, Importance of Chemical Composition of Soybean Products" Journal of Nutrition; 74:587-601.

[7] Potter SM et al., "Soy Protein in Isoflavones, The Effects of Blood Lipids and Bone Density in Postmenopausal Women" American Journal Clin. Nutr. (1998); 68 (6):1375S-1379S.

[8] Aldercreutz H et al., "Excretion of the Lignans Enterolactone and Enterodiol and of Equol in Omnivorous and Vegetarian Postmenopausal Women and in Women with Breast Cancer" Lancet (1982); 2:1295-99.

9 Adlercreutz H et al., "Determinations of the Urinary Lignans and Phytoestrogen Metabolites Potential Antiestrogens and Carcinogens in Urine on Various Habitual Diets" J Steroid Biochem (1986):25791-797.

10 We et al., "Carcinogenesis" (Sept. 2002)

11 (Sept. 2002) Cancer Epidemiology, Biomarkers & Prevention

12 Xu X, Duncan AM et al., "Effects of Soy Isoflavones on Estrogen and Phytoestrogen Metabolism in Premenopausal Women" Cancer Epidemiology Biomarkers & Prevention (1998) 7 (12):1101-08.

13 Lee John R "What Your Doctor May Not Tell You About Breast Cancer" Warner Books (2002):252-253.

14 Arnot R "The Breast Cancer Prevention Diet" Little Brown (1998):59.

8

Black Cohosh: Natures Symptom Fighter

Black Cohosh (Cimicifuga racemosa) is a plant native to North America. It was used by Native Americans for a variety of ailments, including menstrual problems, arthritis, snake bites and kidney ailments. The root of this plant contains phytoestrogens, including formononetin (an Isoflavone) and 27-deoxyactein (a triterpenoid glycoside).[7] Formononetin and 27-deoxyactein have been shown to have an affinity for estrogen receptors. Like the Isoflavones we talked about in Chapter Seven (soy and flax) the phytoestrogens from Black Cohosh attach to the estrogen receptors and exert a mild estrogenic effect.

Black Cohosh has been approved by the German Ministry of Health (Kommission E) and has been one of the most prescribed herbs in Germany for several decades. For those of you who are not familiar with Kommission E, it is an FDA-like body that evaluates nutrients and supplements for effectiveness and possible toxicity. It then approves or rejects them for use by the German public.

Many studies have shown Black Cohosh is effective in treating the symptoms associated with menopause. These studies include the following:

Study 1 629 women were given a liquid extract of Black Cohosh, 40 drops twice per day for 6-8 weeks. 80% of the women had significant improvement in menopausal symptoms by the end of the study. Black

Cohosh was well tolerated. No one was forced to quit the study due to side effects and only 7% of people reported stomach upset, which resolved. [2] (To review symptom by symptom, please see Figure 8A.)

Figure 8A

Symptom	% No Longer Present	% Improved	Total Improved
Hot Flashes	43.3%	43.3%	86.6%
Profuse Sweating	49.9%	38.6%	88.5%
Headache	45.7%	36.2%	81.9%
Vertigo	51.6%	35.2%	86.8%
Heart Palpitations	54.6%	35.2%	90.4%
Ear Ringing	54.8%	38.1%	92.9%
Nervousness/ Irritability	42.4%	43.2%	85.6%
Sleep disturbances	46.1%	30.7%	76.8%
Depressive moods	46.0%	36.5%	82.5%

Ref 2

You will note from this study that even difficult to control symptoms, such as vertigo and heart palpitations improved by nearly 90% with over 50% of the women having complete resolution of all symptoms of menopause.

Study 2 60 women were given either standardized Black Cohosh extract, Valium (2 mg a day) or conjugated estrogen (0.625 mg a day) for 12 weeks. Black Cohosh was shown to be more effective for the relief of depression and anxiety related to menopause than either

Valium or conjugated estrogen 0.625. Results were measured by the Kupperman Menopause Index. [3] (Figure 8B.)

Figure 8B

	Before Treatment	After Treatment
Black Cohosh	35	14
Conjugated Estrogen	35	16
Diazepam (Valium)	35	20

Study 3 In this study of 80 women, Black Cohosh was compared with conjugated estrogen 0.625 mg and placebo. 30 women took Black Cohosh, 2 tablets of standardized extract twice per day, and 30 women took conjugated estrogen 0.625 mg daily, and 20 took placebo. Symptoms improved more dramatically in the Black Cohosh group vs the conjugated estrogen group. As an example, hot flashes dropped from an average of 5 per day to less than 1 per day in the Black Cohosh group vs 5 per day reducing to 3.5 per day in the conjugated estrogen group. This study also showed that Black Cohosh was able to improve vaginal cell proliferation.[4] The author states that "Black Cohosh outperformed conjugated estrogen in this study". Author's note: We have discussed before that improvement in vaginal cell proliferation improves the elasticity in the vagina reducing pain with intercourse and allowing for more normal vaginal function.

Study 4 A double blind study done on 110 women compared Black Cohosh vs placebo. Black Cohosh improved nervousness, hot flashes and night sweats. Women took either 2 mg of standardized Black Cohosh extract twice daily or placebo for two months. Interestingly enough, not only did symptoms improve, but serum levels of LH (luteinizing hormone) went down. FSH (follicle stimulating hormone) was unchanged.[6] Scientists have believed that rising levels of luteinizing hormone (LH) are responsible for causing hot flashes and night sweats. The fact that Black Cohosh has the ability to lower LH suggests that this may be one of the mechanisms responsible for Black Cohosh's ability to reduce hot flashes.

Study 5 60 women under the age of 40 were placed on 1 of 4 treatments. All of the women in this study had one ovary or part of an ovary removed and were having significant menopausal symptoms. The women were divided into four groups.

1) Group 1 were given Black Cohosh, 2 tablets of standarized extract twice daily.
2) Group 2 were given Estriol, 1 mg daily.
3) Group 3 were given conjugated estrogens, 1.25 mg daily.
4) Group 4 were given estrogen and progesterone combination, 1 tablet daily (Trisequens).

The estrogen hormones did lower the Kupperman Index more than the Black Cohosh, yet this study shows Black Cohosh was effective in relieving the symptoms of partial oophorectomy (removal of an ovary).[5]

Discussion

These studies demonstrate Black Cohosh's ability to reduce menopausal symptoms as well as or better than 0.625 mg of conjugated estrogen, in most cases, without evidence of serious side effect. The most serious side effect was nausea and stomach upset, which in most cases was transient. A six month chronic toxicity study in rats at nearly 90 times the human therapeutic dose, showed no toxic effect.[6] Black Cohosh has been used by thousands of women in Germany and around the world since the 1950's. No reports of serious side effects have been noted. Let's discuss, however, several important precautions:

1) Never use Black Cohosh if you are pregnant or breast-feeding. (Although it is not known if Black Cohosh would be toxic or dangerous. No studies have been done to confirm its safety in pregnancy or breast-feeding.)
2) Never use black Cohosh if you are allergic to aspirin. Black Cohosh contains salicylic acid and may react if you are allergic to aspirin.
3) Always use a standardized extract of a brand name Black Cohosh. It should be standardized to 1 mg of 27-deoxyactein per tablet. It is vital that you use the highest quality herb and/or supplements available. The industry has multiple ways of deceiving you. Not all products are the same. Some contain very poor quality supplements that are lower than listed in active ingredients or may contain no active ingredients whatsoever! Other products contain chemicals and/or racemic mixtures that could be harmful to your health. Remember, there is no regulatory agency monitoring the purity of supplements. Therefore buyers beware. You should always use a brand that you know and trust. In the case of herbs, always use standardized products. Throughout this book, when I discuss nutrients and/or supplements, especially herbs, I will

list for you the standardized dose and try to alert you to the most common mistakes people make when purchasing supplements. (In the back of this book is a product section that contains the supplements and/or herbs that I have used in the clinic to obtain the desired results.)

Summary

Black Cohosh is a plant, the root of which contains substances that are phytoestrogens and have been used for centuries by Native Americans. It has been used as a standardized herbal therapy since roughly the 1950's throughout Europe. Many studies have shown Black Cohosh to be as effective in relieving menopausal symptoms as low to moderate doses of conjugated estrogens. Studies have shown Black Cohosh apparently does not increase the risk of breast cancer as opposed to estrogen replacement therapy. While side effects are not impossible with Black Cohosh, they are, for the most part, rare and mild. They include nausea and breast tenderness. These symptoms usually resolve with reducing the dose and/or discontinuance of the product. You should take the lowest dose of standardized extract that relieves your menopausal symptoms, and as always, do so under the supervision of an appropriate health care practitioner. If your menopausal symptoms are well controlled using Black Cohosh as a supplement, you should work to prevent osteoporosis since the studies are not conclusive that Black Cohosh protects bone. Many experts believe that it does reduce bone destruction, but this has not been proven. Your calcium intake should be 2000 mg or more per day (of absorbable calcium). You must have adequate vitamin D intake of 400 – 800 IU daily, along with the other essential minerals necessary to maintain your bone strength, including Magnesium and Boron.

Overdose

Symptoms of overdose include headache, nausea, vomiting, dizziness, visual and nervous disturbances, breast tenderness, reduced pulse rate and increased perspiration. [7] If you have these symptoms, reduce or discontinue Black Cohosh immediately.

Black Cohosh has been a safe, effective therapy for controlling menopausal symptoms. It does not appear to carry the risks associated with estrogen replacement therapy (ERT), and has been used by millions of women throughout the world to improve their quality of life. No supplement, herb, or drug is without possible side effects, but Black Cohosh has shown a low side effect profile with minor symptoms of nausea and breast tenderness in a small percentage of the women studied (approximately 7%). In these studies, even the minor symptoms or side effects appear to be self-limiting.

As we discussed in the last chapter, if you have menopausal symptoms the place to start is with your diet. Increase the soy and flax phytoestrogens in your diet to see if you can control your symptoms. If you cannot and need a supplement to improve your quality of life, then consideration can be made for standardized Black Cohosh in addition to your dietary changes. Use the lowest dose of Black Cohosh that controls your symptoms. Through this plan, many of you will be able to avoid estrogen replacement therapy (ERT) altogether and avoid the risks associated with ERT. Obviously, if you are on a supplement of Black Cohosh, continue to get your yearly breast checks, mammograms and Pap smears (or more frequently as advised by your personal physician). Most physicians have no knowledge of Black Cohosh. Unfortunately, many physicians instead of learning about the benefits of Black Cohosh will belittle you for taking it. I never recommend hiding any supplement program from your physician. However, if your physician belittles you for taking Black Cohosh, then it is time to find a new physician. The days of making the patient feel foolish because the doctor is ignorant of natural or nutritional therapy are over.

Let's go on and talk about another hormone that is very important in reducing your breast cancer risk. This is the "Cinderella of hormones" since it is neglected and abused by so many physicians, yet has the power to help prevent bone loss, control many perimenopausal symptoms and reduce your breast cancer risk. What is this "Cinderella hormone?" PROGESTERONE......

---

[2] Stolze H "An Alternative to Treat Menopausal Complaints" Gynecology 3 (1982):14-16.
[3] Warnecki G "Influencing Menopause Symptoms with a Thytotherapeutic Agent" Medizinische Welt 36 (1985):626-9.
[4] Stoll W "Phytopharmacon Influences Atrophic Vaginal Epithelium. Double-Blind Study- Cimicifuga vs Estrogenic Substances" Therapeuticum (1987):23-31.
[5] Lehman-Willenbrock E. "Clinical and Endocrinologic Examinations of Climacteric Symptoms Following Hysterectomy with Remaining Ovaries" Zentrallbatt für Gynakologie 110 (10) 1988:611-618.
[6] Murray Michael T "Ask the Doctor" Vital Communications Inc. (1997)
[7] LaValle JB "Black Cohosh: A Natural Alternative Method for Balancing Hormone Levels." Avery Press (2000):19.

9

Progesterone: The "Cinderella of Hormones"

Progesterone is a hormone that does not receive the respect from the medical community that it is due. When you are premenopausal, progesterone is made in the ovaries and your levels go up significantly the last two weeks of your cycle. If your body recognizes that you are not pregnant, progesterone levels drop dramatically triggering your period. Most women make, on average, 15-20 mg of progesterone daily, the majority produced in the last two weeks of your cycle. [1] Progesterone goes through your bloodstream where it exerts its effect on many organs including the uterus, breasts and brain just to name a few. Most doctors forget that progesterone affects multiple organs, not just the uterus. In the brain it has calming antidepressant-like effects and seems to help with sleep. In the breasts, it helps prevent overstimulation by estrogen. In the skeletal system, it acts to increase bone formation allowing a woman to actively build bone. Remember, estrogen does not help you to build bone, it slows the breakdown of bone. This breakdown is called osteoclastic activity. It is important to realize that progesterone has a whole host of actions in the body, beyond just getting the uterus ready for conception and/or maintaining a pregnancy. In the clinic I have seen hundreds of women who have had a total hysterectomy (ovaries and uterus removed), and they are just on estrogen replacement therapy (ERT). The gynecologists believe that because you no longer have a uterus, you no longer need progesterone. Nothing could be further from the truth! I suppose this is understandable, since your gynecologist is just thinking about your reproductive system. However, it is still inexcusable. All doctors must consider the effects of their therapy throughout the body not just on one organ system. I have had many hundreds of patients who had resolution of their migraines, fibrocystic breasts, anxiety and improvement of their libido once they started on natural bioidentical progesterone. The crazy thing about it is that many of these patients had gone to their gynecologist, prior to seeing me, complaining of these exact symptoms. They were prescribed an antidepressant and were told they were depressed! Unfortunately, ignorance is not bliss when it is <u>your</u> body that has to go without progesterone. <u>IMPORTANT POINT:</u> If you have had a total hysterectomy, you still need <u>progesterone!</u> (For the type and dose, see the end of the chapter.)

In addition, I have seen many symptomatic women (with intact ovaries) in their 30's or early 40's who are not low in estrogen, but are low in progesterone. There are several reasons for this:

1) By the age of 35 approximately 50% of women have dysfunctional follicles leading to cycles where they do not ovulate or luteal insufficiency (the corpus luteum is the structure in the ovaries that produces progesterone after you ovulate).[1] If you are one of these women who either do not ovulate or have dysfunctional follicles, you will be low in progesterone with its associated symptoms.

2) Stress. In times of high stress the body is able to take progesterone and remove one small side group to make it into cortisone. When you are under stress cortisone becomes the more important hormone. You need higher levels of cortisone to handle either psychological or physical stress. If the stress continues for a prolonged period of time, progesterone levels start to go down causing associated symptoms. This has one evolutionary advantage in that if your progesterone levels drop

significantly, you will not make the progesterone necessary to maintain a pregnancy. Think about this for a minute. In the not so distant past, prolonged stress was from war, famine, or severe prolonged weather changes. This is not exactly a great time to have a baby, so the body accomplishes two goals with one stone. You get more cortisone, which you need in times of stress and it becomes harder for you to become pregnant (which you do not need during war or famine). Let's look at what happens in the 21st Century. Stresses are no longer war, famine or disease (at least for those of us in the Western world). More than likely your stresses are job stresses, divorce, law suits, traffic jams and financial problems just to name a few. Some of you may stay under severe stress for many years. The average divorce is 2-3 years in length. An even bigger problem is long-term job stress and/or family distress. These stresses last for decades and slowly wear down your adrenal glands. The adrenal glands are small glands at the top of our kidneys where we make over 100 hormones, including cortisone and DHEA. After menopause, these glands are responsible for making estrogen and progesterone since your ovaries are no longer functioning or functioning in a reduced capacity. If you wear down your adrenals, you are no longer able to produce the cortisone necessary to handle stress. Your body then pulls progesterone into the cortisol pathway to try to compensate and you are left with chronically low progesterone levels (this assumes that your ovaries are functioning properly). This is a big assumption since most women who have worn down adrenal function also have ovarian dysfunction. Many of you reading this right now are low in progesterone since it is the most common sex hormone deficiency in a pre-menopausal woman. Symptoms of progesterone deficiency can include irregular periods, fibrocystic breast disease, anxiety, depression, mood swings particularly prior to menses, difficulty thinking and more.

What Does all this have to do with Breast Cancer?

Progesterone is vital to balancing the stimulatory effects of estrogen in the breasts. We already have talked at length about how estrogen (with the exception of Estriol) strongly stimulates breast tissue cellular reproduction. The higher your strong estrogen levels the more rapidly your breast tissue will reproduce and the thicker and larger your breasts become, eventually developing fibrocysts. If this cellular reproduction is not controlled you could develop a tumor (i.e. cancer). We have discussed the fact that estrogen is vital in keeping your breast tissue young, firm, and healthy (among its many other benefits). THE KEY IS BALANCE! Progesterone was designed to balance out the stimulatory effects of estrogen in the breast and elsewhere. Progesterone does so through the following mechanisms:

1) Progesterone decreases the cellular levels of estrogen receptors. This reduces breast cells response to the stimulatory effects of estrogens. [1]

2) Progesterone increases conversions of estrogen to inactive sulfate. [1]

3) Progesterone increases thyroid activity, which increases sulfotransferase and SHBG (sex hormone binding globulin). This lowers the amount of available estrogen. [1]

4) Progesterone blocks the formation of cancer causing catechol estrogen. [1]

5) Progesterone lowers the level of prolactin, a tumor growth promoter. [1]

6) Progesterone reduces breast cell uptake of Estradiol. [1]

Research has shown that women who are low in progesterone are at a greater risk of breast cancer and are twice as likely to die of that breast cancer as a woman with normal progesterone levels. A study published in The American Journal of Epidemiology in 1981 showed that women who were deficient in progesterone were over 5 times as likely to get breast cancer as those with normal progesterone levels. [2]

A 1998 study published in The Annals of Clinical and Laboratory Science found that in T47-D cancer cells the p53 gene was upregulated by progesterone.[3] (The p53 is a tumor suppressor gene which improves apoptosis-programmed cell death for abnormal cancer cells.)

Summary

Progesterone is the "Cinderella of Hormones", as it has too often been ignored or dismissed. We have briefly reviewed some of the evidence that shows it is important in preventing breast cancer. The study published in The American Journal of Epidemiology showed women who were deficient in progesterone were 5 times as likely to get breast cancer as women who were not. Not only is progesterone protective for the breasts, but it has therapeutic effects throughout the body including stabilizing and calming the nervous system, encouraging bone production, protecting and/or encouraging thyroid function, and energy production. Millions of you who have had a total hysterectomy have been told you have no need for progesterone. I hope you see by now, nothing could be further from the truth. If your progesterone levels are low (since your ovaries are removed we assume they are low) progesterone supplementation is indicated.

How Do we Measure Progesterone Levels?

The best way to measure progesterone is through saliva. We are measuring free progesterone levels and it is this free hormone that has the ability to exert its effect. Salivary measurements are an excellent way of measuring nearly all hormones, since it gives the free hormone levels, which as stated above, are the hormones that are active. Many hormones are protein bound or bound to binding substances such as SHBG (sex hormone binding globulin), which binds estrogen and/or progesterone and does not allow it to exert its effect. In addition, saliva allows us to obtain levels at several different times during the cycle improving accuracy. Remember you make the majority of progesterone the last two weeks of your cycle. This is when progesterone should be measured. Millions of you have had serum progesterone levels done, which in many cases have been normal. You have been told your progesterone levels are normal. Serum progesterone, however, evaluates the bound and unbound hormone and does not give an accurate reflection of your true free hormone status.

What Type of Progesterone Supplementation is Best?

ALWAYS use natural bioidentical progesterone.* Most doctors prescribe synthetic progestins, which are not progesterone. Progestins are progesterone-like hormones that exert progesterone-like effects in some instances, but in other instances have effects different than progesterone. One of the problems has been that progesterone is a natural substance and cannot be patented; therefore, a pharmaceutical company cannot hold the absolute unchallenged patent on progesterone. For this reason, pharmaceutical companies developed progestins, which are substances that mimic progesterone, but are not the same hormone. Studies now are showing that progestins may increase the risk of breast cancer. These studies include the recent Women's Health Initiative (WHI), which showed that women on a conjugated estrogen/synthetic progestin had a significant increase in their risk of breast cancer. Your doctor, including most gynecologists, may not be familiar with natural progesterone. One piece of good news is that oral progesterone has been released by a major pharmaceutical company in tablet form. Therefore, many physicians are becoming

*Bioidentical means that the progesterone in the supplement has the identical structure as human progesterone.

familiar with progesterone through that pharmaceutical company. The problem is that you should never take oral progesterone unless absolutely necessary. As we discussed with estrogen, progesterone cream is well absorbed, therefore, you are able to use lower doses than oral progesterone. Oral progesterone has to be given in much higher doses with a large percentage of it being converted to metabolites. This does not make sense to me. If you are going to take progesterone, make sure it is natural bioidentical progesterone and make sure it is progesterone cream. Start off with a low dose, 12.5 mg or possibly less, and titrate up if you do not get control of your symptoms. If you are a pre-menopausal woman, with intact ovaries and uterus, we give progesterone cream the last two weeks of the cycle to more closely mimic what you would produce naturally. The doses can range between 6 mg and 100 mg (average dose is 12.5 – 25 mg). Usually the higher doses are reserved for those women with very severe PMS. If you are a post-menopausal woman, you need lower amounts of progesterone to mimic what the body would normally produce after menopause. You can take progesterone daily, in smaller amounts usually 6-25 mg. As I discussed in the Estriol chapter, if you are on Estriol cream progesterone can be built right into the same cream. This will reduce your cost and also reduce the hassle.

Possible Side Effects

The major side effect from progesterone, if you have an intact uterus, and take too much progesterone is early or prolonged menstrual bleeding (bleeding in between periods). If this happens, slowly reduce the dose of progesterone to eliminate that side effect. Most women find progesterone helpful for fibrocystic disease. I have had 1 or 2 patients who felt it increased their fibrocystic tenderness and they discontinued the progesterone. Many creams are in a soy base. If you are allergic to soy, then creams are available in a non-soy formula.

Progesterone creams

Progesterone creams can be made by a competent compounding pharmacist. For further information see the product section at the back of this book.

Studies have shown that women who were deficient in progesterone were at 5 times greater risk of breast cancer than women with normal levels! You must know your progesterone level and if it is low, supplement with a bioidentical progesterone cream. You can monitor your levels by a saliva progesterone study and your health care practitioner can adjust your dose accordingly.

---

[1] Lee JR et al., "What Your Doctor May Not Tell You About Breast Cancer" Warner Books (2002):156.

[2] Cowan LD et al., "Breast Cancer Incidence in Women with a History of Progesterone Deficiency" American Journal of Epidemiology Aug.; 114 (2):209-17 (1981)

[3] Formby B et al., "Progesterone Inhibits Growth and Induces Apoptosis in Breast Cancer cells: Inverse Effects on Bcl-2 and p53" Ann Clin Lab Sci (1998 Nov. – Dec.); 28 (6):360-69

10

The Super Vitamin E That Can Reduce Breast Cancer

Vitamin E is one of the most important fat soluble antioxidants in our body. Since breasts are predominantly fat, it would make sense that vitamin E could reduce oxidative damage to breast tissue, therefore, reducing the risk of breast cancer. But, is this true? Do medical studies support the fact that vitamin E reduces breast cancer risks? Let's look at the studies.

An interesting observation has been made over the last several years. Studies done on women who eat foods high in vitamin E suggests they have a significant reduction in their breast cancer risk, yet women taking vitamin E supplements, sometimes at several hundred times the dose that you would get from your diet, did not reduce their risk of cancer at all. [1,2] What is going on here? To answer that let's first review the studies done on the total vitamin E intake and reduction of breast cancer risks since those studies are rather compelling.

1) If you are premenopausal with a family history of breast cancer, and you are in the group of women with the highest vitamin E levels, you have a 90% reduction of your risk of breast cancer.1,

2) If you are a premenopausal woman without a family history of breast cancer, and are in the group with the highest levels of vitamin E you have a 50% risk reduction. 1

3) If you are a postmenopausal woman without a family history of breast cancer and you are in the group that is highest in vitamin E, you have a 50% reduction of breast cancer risk. [1]

4) Lastly, if you are a postmenopausal woman with a family history of breast cancer, and you are in the group highest in vitamin E, you still have a 30% reduction of risk.[1]

5) This remarkable study shows that if you obtain high levels of vitamin E at a younger age, you can achieve a 90% reduction in your breast cancer risk, even if you have a positive family history. (Author's Note: This is just with vitamin E alone, not including all of the other risk reducing secrets we have discussed.) Importantly, it also shows that it is never too late, since even postmenopausal women had a 30-50% reduction in their breast cancer risk. This study is truly amazing! Remember, however, this was total vitamin E from dietary sources. Studies done on alpha tocopherol acetate are much less compelling. (Author's Note: Alpha tocopherol is the type of vitamin E usually found in vitamin E supplements.) In fact, many of these studies failed to show significant risk reduction at all with vitamin E supplement. [1,2,4,5]

How can this be? It is important to remember vitamin E is not just one vitamin; it is a family with multiple different members. Alpha tocopherol was the first member of the vitamin E family discovered; therefore was given the name vitamin E. For many decades doctors thought it was that simple. Vitamin E was alpha tocopherol. What they did not know and what we know now is there is not only alpha tocopherol, but beta, delta and gamma. All of these tocopherols, plus the tocotrienols (beta, delta and gamma) make up what we now know as vitamin E. These substances work as a team and occur together in nature in the same foods. That is why when you take commercially available vitamin E supplements, in most cases, you are getting just a small fraction of the true benefits of vitamin E complex. An example would be: A football coach hiring a quarterback, but not bothering to hire any blockers or receivers. It is nice to have a quarterback, but without other qualified team members you are not getting the maximal result. The same principal applies with vitamin E. You need the whole team to get the true benefits from vitamin E.

Let's talk for a few minutes about the vitamin E cousins named tocotrienols. I hope you will be as impressed with this information as I was when I first reviewed it.

In several studies tocotrienols were shown to slow the growth of estrogen receptor positive breast cancer cells (in culture) by up to 50%.[6,7] Some studies have shown that tocotrienols also work on estrogen receptor negative (ER negative) breast cancer. Tocotrienols appear to accomplish this by restoring the ability of the breast cancer cells to self-destruct. All cells have a mechanism that allows them to self-destruct if they become too damaged or abnormal. The concept is: Cancer cells lose their ability for self destruction. Even though they are very abnormal, they continue to reproduce, eventually building up enough numbers to cause a tumor. If this self destructive mechanism was maintained, as it is in normal cells, the cells would detect that they had become significantly abnormal and self-destruct. Tocotrienols help to restore breast cancer cells self destruction (apoptosis).[8] One study took different types of live breast cancer cells and injected them into the mammary tissue of female mice. Tocotrienols were found to inhibit the growth of each of the breast cancer cell lines tested.[7] It is not surprising that studies have shown that regular vitamin E supplements (alpha tocopherol) do not appear to reduce the risk of breast cancer, yet <u>vitamin E complex</u>, including the "cousins" named tocotrienols, have been shown to significantly reduce the risk of breast cancer and restore breast cancer cells ability to self-destruct. This is why studies showing vitamin E obtained from the diet significantly reduced the risk of breast cancer in premenopausal and postmenopausal women alike. The vitamin E that is obtained from the diet is the complete vitamin E complex. (As we have already discussed, all of these vitamin E family members hang around together in the same food.)

It is interesting to note that the Standard American Diet (SAD) contains very little vitamin E. Most vitamin E occurs in whole grains, particularly the GERM of the grain. The GERM is the part of the grain that can sprout, with the remainder of the kernel being mostly starch to feed the new sprout once it develops. The germ is the part of the kernel, be it wheat, corn or any other grain that is highest in oil. As you all know, oil can turn rancid if left on the shelf for long periods of time. Beginning roughly in the mid-20th Century, food companies figured out that if they removed the GERM from the grain, the bread would last much longer on the shelf. Prior to that, most breads were made with whole grain and once baked would last only for several days. (Author's Note: Many of you remember, as I do, day-old-bread being half off at our local bakery. The reason for that was, the bread spoiled more quickly with the whole grain containing the GERM than bread where the GERM had been removed and preservatives added. As a poor college student, I once kept a loaf of bread on my shelf for two months without it spoiling! The name of this bread is being withheld to protect the not-so-innocent.) Food companies removed the GERM and replaced it with the newly discovered vitamin E, thinking they were replacing some of the same nutrients that they removed. Remember, this vitamin E was just alpha tocopherol, since no one knew that vitamin E was an entire family. They call this bread enriched! As my father used to say, "That is like taking a dollar from you, giving you 7 cents back and telling you that you are now enriched!" Another interesting fact from my father, when mice get into the corn crib and can eat any part of the corn they please, all they eat is the GERM. They leave the remainder of the kernel, the part that contains mostly starch. Do you think nature is trying to tell us something? If mice know enough to just eat the GERM and you are several hundred times smarter than a mouse, then what is your excuse for eating the part of the kernel that even a mouse will not eat? The answer to this is mice know that the GERM contains the majority of nutrients, oils, and antioxidants that are important for health. In addition, the mice do not have food companies preparing their foods nor do they have to watch the endless stream of advertisements selling foods that are not very beneficial to health. This is not just true for corn, but, wheat, rice, and all grains have had the GERM removed, unless they are "whole". (When you eat white rice the rice bran and GERM has been removed; therefore, very little vitamin E or tocotrienol remains. To get the true benefit from rice you would have to eat natural whole rice.)

Tocotrienol supplements are usually made from rice bran or palm oil. Since tocotrienols are fat soluble, your breasts tend to concentrate much higher levels than your blood. Since tocotrienols (the entire vitamin E family) are fat soluble, they do not wash out of the body as easy as water soluble vitamins. Vitamin E is stored in your fat; therefore, eating small amounts of foods containing the vitamin E family every day may pay huge benefits. (See figure 10A.)

Foods High in Vitamin E	IU
Wheat germ 2 tbs	20.0
Almonds 1 ounce	7.5
Whole grain bread (slice)	1-3 IU
Rice Bran (100 gm)	45 IU
Mango	2.3
Filberts	20 IU
Sunflower Seeds 2 tbs	10 IU
Shrimp 3 ounces	≈ 5-7 IU
Broccoli ½ cup	1.5
Spinach ½ cup	≈ 1.0
Quick Tip Easy tip to increase the Vitamin E in your diet is to add 2 tablespoons of organic wheat germ to your favorite cereal (hot or cold) or add it to your flax muffin recipe. Wheat allergy is the third most common allergy in the U.S. Avoid wheat germ if you suspect you are allergic to wheat.	

Figure 10A

If you want to use a supplement, what should you look for?

1) Never take a vitamin E that is just alpha tocopherol.

2) You should always supplement with a vitamin E that contains the whole family. Mixed tocopherols plus tocotrienols.

3) You can overdose on vitamin E because it is fat soluble, but you have to try fairly hard. Several studies have shown 240 mg per day of tocotrienols for 16 months produced no adverse side effects.[7] This study also showed that supplementation of 78 mg of tocotrienols for one month produced an eight-fold increase in blood levels. These blood levels approximated the level that was found to slow estrogen receptor positive breast cancer cell division by 50%.[7]

4) Other studies have shown gamma tocopherol and possibly tocotrienols to be COX-2 inhibitors. [9] COX-2 enzyme has been shown to be involved in the development of cancer. As we will discuss in later chapters, inhibition or reduction of the COX-2 enzyme, reduces cancer risk.

Summary

1) The vitamin E family has been shown to reduce the risk of breast cancer from 50-90% in premenopausal and 30-50% in postmenopausal women.

2) The vitamin E family consists of many members, not just alpha tocopherol. Alpha tocopherol is the type of vitamin E that is in most commercial vitamin E supplements.

3) You should immediately increase the foods that are high in vitamin E content. (See Table 10A.)

4) Supplementation of a complete vitamin E complex makes sense for most women. As we have discussed, make sure your supplement contains mixed tocopherols plus tocotrienols. (Author's note: Be careful. Some supplements will say with mixed tocopherols, but when you read the label only a small fraction of the total E is beta, delta and gamma. For the vitamin E supplement I recommend see the products section in the back of this book.)

5) Dose. 100 to 800 IU daily.

6) Vitamin E supplements should be taken with meals since they are oil based and require some fat in our food to be effectively absorbed.

7) Caution: If you are on blood thinning medications, such as Coumadin™ (Warfarin) or Heparin, vitamin E may increase the effect. Always consult with your physician prior to starting vitamin E supplementation if you are on blood thinning medications. Vitamin E is very beneficial for cardiovascular disease. In most cases one can take a vitamin E supplement if they are on blood thinning medications, as long as those

medication levels are monitored with adjustment in the dose as indicated.

We have kept our discussion of vitamin E restricted to its benefits in reducing breast cancer. Of course, you have fat in many other areas of your body and the benefits from mixed vitamin E supplementation include: cardiovascular risk reduction, reduction in inflammation, slowing of the aging process and reduction of the risk of several other cancers. This is one of those simple secrets you can use to dramatically reduce your risk of breast cancer! The information that we have reviewed concerning tocotrienols is truly cutting-edge. You may not read about it in newspapers or the popular press for years. Your doctor may not know about it for decades. You now have this dramatic information which you can use to significantly reduce your breast cancer risk. Vitamin E complex supplementation is part of an overall breast cancer reduction plan that can dramatically reduce the chances of you ever hearing those dreaded words, "YOU HAVE BREAST CANCER."

---

[1] Freudenheim J.L. et al., "Premenopausal Breast Cancer Risk and Intake of Vegetables, Fruits and Related Nutrients," Journal of National Cancer Institute 88 (1996):340-348.

[2] Hunter D.J. et al, "A Prospective Study of the Intake of Vitamin C, Vitamin E and Vitamin A, and the Risk of Breast Cancer.," New England Journal of Medicine 329 (1993):234-40.

[1] Ambrosine C.B. et al., "Interaction of Family History of Breast Cancer and Dietary Antioxidants with
Breast Cancer Risk," Cancer: Causes & Control 6 (1995): 407-415.

[4] Zhong S. et al., "Dietary Carotenoids and Vitamin C, A, and E and Risk of Breast Cancer," Journal of National Cancer Institute 91 (1999):547-56.

[5] Rohan T.E. et al., "Dietary Fiber, Vitamin A, C, E and Risk of Breast Cancer Cohort Study," Cancer,
Causes and Control 4 (1993):29-37.

[6] Nesaretnam K et al., "Tocotrienols Inhibit the Growth of Human Breast Cancer Cells Irrespective of
Estrogen Receptor Status," Lipids 33 (1998): 461-69.

[7] Morrow Michele, M.D., "Does Vitamin E Prevent Breast Cancer?" Life Extension (May 2002): 29-35.
[8] Yu W. et al., "Induction of Apoptosis in Human Breast Cancer Cells by Tocopherols and Tocotrienols," Nutr Cancer 33 (1999): 26-32.
[9] Turley J.M. et al., "Vitamin E Succinate Inhibits Proliferation of BT-20 Human Breast Cancer Cells," Cancer Research 57/13 (1997):2668-75.

11

Curcumin:
Natures Anticancer "Secret Agent"

- Curcumin is the active ingredient in Tumeric. Tumeric is a yellow/orange spice from the root of the plant Curcuma longa. Curcuma longa is a plant similar to ginger that grows in tropical areas. Tumeric has been used in the ancient medicines of India and China for nearly 6000 years. Many ancient texts have described the anti-inflammatory properties of Tumeric. It has been used for the treatment of various diseases including arthritis and bowel dysfunction. Tumeric is more than likely one of those substances that began as a medicine and eventually evolved into a ubiquitous part of the cultures diet. Many recipes from India contain Tumeric. This accomplishes two goals: 1) it helps with taste. 2) It is an anti-inflammatory medication.
- Curcumin can block chemicals like DDT and dioxin from getting inside your breast cells. It does this by attaching itself to the "Ah" receptor. This is the receptor that DDT and dioxin use to gain access to your breast cells. (Remember in the chapter on I3C and DIM we discussed the "Ah" receptor since I3C and DIM also competitively inhibit dioxin and DDT from attaching to the "Ah" receptor and triggering uncontrollable breast cell reproduction). In one study, curcumin reduced DDT's ability to cause growth of breast cancer by 75%.[4]

- Curcumin has also been shown to block other cancer causing chemicals including pesticides. [10,4]
- Liver cancer dropped from 100% to 38% in mice given both curcumin and a known cancer causing chemical. [7,12]
- Curcumin not only helps protect your breast cells from harmful chemicals, but also from radiation. Rats irradiated to produce breast cancer were given curcumin. The group given the curcumin had an 18.55% risk of developing breast cancer vs 70% for those rats who did not receive curcumin. [2] A Japanese study confirms the amazing finding that 85% of irradiated rats got breast cancer vs 28% for the group that received curcumin and radiation. [3]
- Curcumin reversed estrogen induced growth of breast cancer cells by 98%![4]
- Studies have shown breast tumor cell lines are sensitive to curcumin even when they may be resistant to all known drugs.[5]

How can curcumin have such a dramatic protectant effect on breast cells, yet a devastating effect on breast cancer?

1) Curcumin blocks breast cancer growth factors, including those named kinase. Curcumin interferes with those signals, therefore, slowing breast cancer growth rates. [8] Studies have shown the structure of curcumin allows it to inhibit multiple kinases and this may be why curcumin has been found to be helpful in preventing multiple known cancers.
2) Curcumin also causes cancer cells to self-destruct. Remember, in the last chapter on vitamin E we discussed that when cells become abnormal or damaged, they should trigger a self destruction

mechanism known as apoptosis. This is one way the body keeps control over damaged cells, preventing them from reproducing. Cancer cells are able to short circuit apoptosis so abnormal cells can continue to reproduce until they become a dangerous tumor. Curcumin seems to restore the cells ability to recognize that it is damaged; therefore triggering the self-destruct mechanism.[3,9]

3) Curcumin slows the growth of cancer cells in the G-2 stage. [6] (Do not worry about these technical terms such as G-2. It is simply one of the phases that cancer cells go through in order to reproduce. I will explain why this is so significant in the next chapter, when we discuss Tea polyphenols, which helps to block breast cancer reproduction at a separate phase. When you combine these two natural substances you block cancer at two of the major phases required for reproduction.)

4) Curcumin appears to fight breast cancer by improving immunity. This is not surprising since curcumin is known to be a strong antiinflammatory and antioxidant. One study showed animals that were given curcumin had increased levels of cancer fighting immune factors. [7,11]

5) Curcumin also inhibits substances that cause tumors to grow blood vessels. Tumors require more blood than normal cells because of their rapid growth. Tumors obtain this blood supply by producing substances named angiogenesis factors. These angiogenesis factors cause an increase in blood vessels growing into the tumor; therefore allowing the tumor to access the nutrients it needs. Curcumin slows or even inhibits this angiogenesis, not allowing blood vessels to grow into tumors and depriving tumors of the nutrients they need. [6] Without the proper blood supply, tumors

simply cannot continue to grow; therefore, inhibition of angiogenesis is an important factor in controlling the growth rate of the tumor and your survival rate. Currently pharmaceutical companies are actively working at finding angiogenesis inhibiting agents that can be patented. I understand why they are doing this. The neat thing is that nature has provided an angiogenesis inhibiting substance that has been known for roughly 6000 years- CURCUMIN! In addition, very few side effects have been associated with curcumin. It appears to be a very safe, natural spice/medicine/supplement.

Summary

- Curcumin is a strong antioxidant, which allows it to protect breast cells from oxidative damage.

- It binds to the "Ah" receptor, blocking the over stimulatory effects of cancer-causing chemicals.

- It helps cancer cells recognize the fact that they are growing out of control, and reestablishes the self-destruct signal causing the defective cells to self-destruct before they develop into a tumor.

- It appears to improve immunity through improving several immune factors. By improving your immune factors you improve the chances of your immune system recognizing and destroying cancer cells before they go out of control.

- Curcumin is an excellent anti-inflammatory via its reduction of the COX-2 enzyme. It appears to reduce many types of inflammation, including the types of inflammation that can lead to cancer.

- Lastly, it reduces the growth of blood vessels into tumor cells, thereby depriving those cells of the nutrients they need to continue to reproduce. Without these vital nutrients, tumors cannot continue to grow or if they grow their rate of growth is significantly reduced. Hopefully, the rate of growth is slow enough where these tumors do not become life-threatening.

Researchers purposely tried to give rats breast cancer, either through chemical exposure or radiation AND curcumin reduced the incidence of breast cancer from 70% to 18% in one study and from 85% to 28% in another!

If curcumin were a drug and able to be patented, it would be worth billions of dollars. You would be overwhelmed with advertisements proclaiming its virtues. Several large pharmaceutical corporations are racing to develop synthetic forms of curcumin so they can patent them and make them into drugs. You, however, do not have to wait to take advantage of this important nutrient! In my opinion, it would be foolish to wait since the synthetic versions will be vastly more expensive and may not be as effective as natural curcumin. Remember we discussed that vitamin E is a family? Well, Curcumin is a combination of several types of natural Curcumenoids. (A whole family of antioxidant substances.) A synthetic version will contain only one form. Curcumin has developed over thousands of years and has been in human use, as a medication, for nearly 6000 years. This is a very long clinical trial. Ancient people did not continue to use a medication that did not work or caused side effects. Natural Curcumin has a very long track record. In addition, scientific studies now support its use in prevention of many types of cancers and particularly breast cancer. Curcumin is cheap, safe and has a very low side effect profile.

Dose The usual dose is 1 gram 2-3 times a day with food.

Purity Remember, quality and purity matter. There are many tumeric/curcumin supplements on the market, some of which I question their quality and/or purity. No one is routinely evaluating nutritional substances for quality and purity. (Author's Note: Recently legislation has been proposed that will allow the FDA to review nutritional supplements for quality, purity and to make sure the amount that is listed on the label is truly present.) Given questions concerning purity and quality, you should only use a Curcumin product that you know and trust. Since it is difficult for most people to determine what a high quality product is, I have listed the curcumin supplement I use in the clinic at the back of this book.

---

[1] Venkatesan N "Pulmonary Protective Effects of Curcumin Against Paraquat Toxicity" (2000) Life Sci; 66 (2):21-28

[2] The Journal Carcinogenesis (21, October 2000) 10:183541.

[3] The Journal Carcinogenesis (20, June 1999) 6:1011-18.

[4] Life Extension Magazine (July 2002)

[5] Breast Cancer Research Res Treat (April 1999):54 (3):269-78.

[6] Mohan R et al., "Curcuminoids Inhibit the Angiogenic Response" Journal of Biological Chemistry (2000) 275 (14):10:405-412.

[7] Life Extension Magazine (July 2002):29.

[8] Jobin C et al., "Curcumin Blocks Cytokine-Medicated NF- Kappa B Activation" J. Immunol (1999);163:3474-83.

[9] Ciolino HP et al., "Affect of Curcumin on the Aryl Hydrocarbon Receptor and Cytochrome p-450 1A1 in MCF-7 Human Breast Carcinoma Cells" Biochem Pharmacal, 56 (1998):197-206.

[10] Park EJ et al., "Protective Effect of Curcumin in Rat Liver Injury Induced by Carbon Tetrachloride" J. Pharm Pharmacal (2000);52:437-40.

[11] Antony S et al., "Immunomodulatory Activity of Curcumin Immunol Invest" (1999); 28:291-303.

[12] Chaung SE et al., "Curcumin-Containing Diet Inhibits Dimethylnitrosamine-Induced Hepatocarcinogenesis" Carcinogenesis (2000); 21:331-35.

12

Tea:
Nature's Anticancer Secret Agent Too

Tea is perhaps the second most popular drink in the world, behind water. Many positive attributes have been given to tea, particularly green tea. The studies we will review show that tea has anti-cancer effects in animals. The main cancer fighting ingredient of green tea is EGCG (epigallocate-chin 3-gallate). The main cancer fighting ingredients in black tea are polyphenols named theoflavins. Animal studies have shown that the EGCG in green tea has a direct anti-cancer effect by blocking cell reproduction in the G1 phase. [1] Remember in the last chapter, we discussed how curcumin blocks cancer cell reproduction in the G2 phase. We also reviewed that there were at least two major phases in cancer cell reproduction. Researchers at the Sloan-Kettering Cancer Center have shown that EGCG from green tea blocks cancer reproduction at the G1 phase. Curcumin blocked cancer reproduction at the G2 phase. The exciting finding was that the two of these together were much stronger than either one separately. In fact, researchers found that when you added both of these nutrients together, you can reduce the amount by several fold and still get significant cancer-killing effects. This means if you combine the EGCG from green tea with curcumin, your cancer-killing effect is greatly multiplied since you are inhibiting cancer reproduction at two phases rather than one.[1] Another interesting fact is that caffeine appears to be a vital ingredient in tea for promotion of cancer preventing effects.[2] The exact mechanism of why caffeine is important to the cancer preventing effects of tea is still unknown. It appears it is best not to get your tea decaffeinated and perhaps drinking green tea is better than a green tea supplement. There are tradeoffs, however, since a green tea supplement will contain much more EGCG than a cup of green tea. Perhaps the best course would be to have a cup of green tea along with a green tea supplement in conjunction with curcumin?

Summary

This chapter shows that two natural ingredients, EGCG (which is in green tea) and curcumin (which is in the spice tumeric) work in conjunction to reduce the risk of cancer through their action of slowing cellular reproduction. Both of these nutrients have very low possibility of side effects. Green tea contains caffeine, but in low amounts, generally ⅓ to ¼ as much as a cup of coffee, and rarely causes the side effects associated with caffeine (such as tachycardia, nervousness and arrhythmias). One caution would be if you have hypertension and/or cardiac disease, then regular green tea is not for you. You can still consider an EGCG supplement, which would provide some measure of cancer prevention. The side effects from curcumin are very limited and are listed back in Chapter 11. These nutrients can serve as major pieces to your cancer prevention puzzle. When we combine these nutrients along with the other cancer preventing antioxidants and nutrients that we discuss in later chapters, it forms a valuable plan that could reduce your risk of breast cancer by 90% or more. To get the best results it is important to recognize that these nutrients work together as a team. Therefore, building them into your diet where appropriate is always the first step. The addition of supplements may be a second step for those who wish more aggressive cancer prevention strategies. Now, let's go on to talk about a fascinating hormone that recently has been shown to reduce the risk of breast cancer by 35%. That hormone is named Melatonin.

---

[1] Khafifa et al., Carcinogenesis, Volume 19 #3(1998):419-24.
[2] Lin J. K., "Cancer Chemo Prevention by Tea Polyphenols," Proc Natl Sci Counc Volume 24 #1 (2000):1-13.

13

Melatonin: Nature's Cancer Preventing Hormone

Scientists have been both puzzled and fascinated by a study published in The Journal Epidemiology in May 1991. This study showed blind women had half the risk of breast cancer as women who maintained their sight.[1] What in the world can explain this phenomenon? Was genetics the answer? It does not seem likely since this study included women who were not only blind from birth, but also blinded by accident. Was it diet? No. Since these women appear to eat the same diet as women who can see. Another study came out in 2001, in The British Journal of Cancer. In that study, the researchers evaluated 15,000 women who were visually impaired via the Cancer Registry of Norway. 400 of these women were totally blind. It was found that the blind women had a 36% lower risk of breast cancer than women with normal sight.[2] How did they explain this? What does a blind woman have that a woman with sight does not? The answer is a blind woman has higher levels of the hormone melatonin.

Melatonin is a hormone produced in a small gland of the brain named the pineal. We make melatonin from the amino acid tryptophan via the process outlined below.

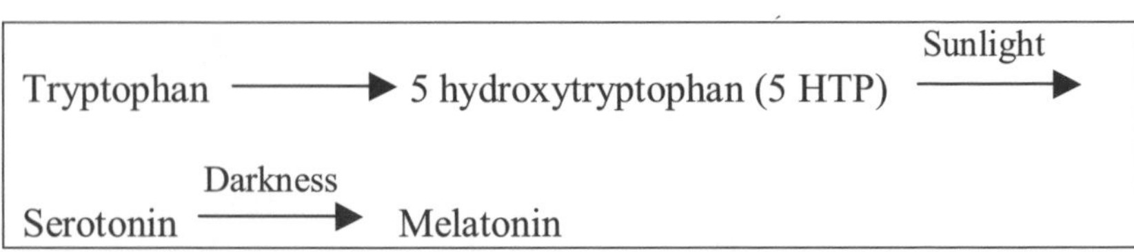

Besides the appropriate enzymes, the other vital ingredient needed to make melatonin is DARKNESS. This is why the blind women had significantly higher levels of melatonin because they are in darkness or near darkness 24 hours a day. This darkness enhances the production of melatonin. The precursor of melatonin, the amino acid Tryptophan is found in turkey, chicken, milk, tuna and soy. It is converted via enzymatic processes to the hormone serotonin, which is associated with improved mood, elevated alertness and excitement. When the sun goes down and we are exposed to darkness serotonin is converted to melatonin. Melatonin we associate with calmness and sleep. As we age, our production of melatonin decreases. Another factor which decreases melatonin is exposure to light in the evening. We will discuss these factors later in this chapter. The big question is why does melatonin so dramatically reduce the risk of breast cancer? The answer lies in the fact that melatonin is a very powerful antioxidant. In fact, melatonin may be the most potent antioxidant in our bodies! Another important factor is that it crosses all known membranes. Therefore, melatonin is both fat and water soluble and able to travel to all cells of the body. When we are young we can make melatonin exceptionally well. (Any of you who have a 5-year-old have seen this in action, since children that age seem to be able to fall asleep instantly.) As we age our ability to make melatonin declines. By age 65, we make only 20-25% the amount of melatonin we made when we were 21. The decrease in production of melatonin seems to begin around age 40 and escalates with age. No one totally understands why melatonin production begins to slow once you are 40. One reason could be that through the years the enzymes that help you to make melatonin have become damaged, therefore, you have trouble converting tryptophan to melatonin. Another reason could be nutritional deficiency. At the clinic we did an unpublished study, which showed 80% of the patients tested were deficient in tryptophan.[3] The cause of this tryptophan deficiency was twofold:

1) As we age, our milk consumption declines, therefore, we just do not eat as many foods that contain tryptophan.

2) A large percentage of people over age 40 have low stomach acid. (Author's Note: I know we have all been told we have too much stomach acid, but the truth is many of you have too little stomach acid.) The amino acid tryptophan requires normal stomach acid levels to be absorbed. If your stomach acid is low, you cannot absorb tryptophan properly, even if you are getting it in your diet. Therefore, less tryptophan less serotonin, less serotonin less melatonin. This may be one reason why so many people in the Western world are depressed. Serotonin is an important anti-depression brain chemical and melatonin is a vital hormone that improves both quantity and quality of sleep. As we have discussed before, one additional cause of low stomach acid is millions of people are taking acid suppression medications. These medications reduce the stomach acid, increase the pH of your stomach and reduce tryptophan absorption.

<u>How Can you Improve your Melatonin Levels?</u>

Giving up your sight to prevent breast cancer seems a little drastic. Let's review what else you can do to improve your levels of melatonin. A couple of studies may shed some "light" on this question. The first study is from <u>The Journal of The National Cancer Institute</u>, which did an analysis of 78,000 women taking part in the Nurses Health Study. The analysis showed that "women who worked up to 29 years on a rotating night shift experienced a moderate increase in breast cancer. Those women who worked over 30 years on rotating night shift had a <u>36% increase</u> in their breast cancer risk."[5] The other study, published again in The Journal of the National Cancer Institute showed that women who did not sleep from 1 a.m. to 2 a.m. had an elevated risk of breast cancer. [4,5] Interpretation: The first study showed that people, who work third shift, even on a rotating basis, make lower amounts of melatonin. Even though their bodies will make some melatonin during the day while they are asleep, they never really produce the amounts that would be expected from someone who sleeps at night. The second study confirms what has been known about melatonin production: we seem to make most of our melatonin (or a bolus of melatonin) between 1 a.m. and 2 a.m. If you are not asleep at 1:00 a.m. you lose a significant amount of your melatonin production, even if you still get a full 8 hours sleep. This reduction in melatonin contributes to poor quality sleep, reduced immunity and reduced antioxidant function. Any of these effects or a combination of the above can contribute to increasing your breast cancer risk.

What Can You Do to Improve Melatonin Production and Decrease your Breast Cancer Risk?

1) Make sure you are asleep before 1 a.m.

2) Eat foods that are high in tryptophan. (That is why your grandmother said to have a glass of warm milk at bedtime. She did not know the medical reasons she just knew that warm milk helped you to fall asleep. That is due to the amino acid tryptophan.) Millions of you are allergic to milk and if you are, you can use soy products and increase your consumption of turkey, preferably at supper. Turkey being high in tryptophan can cause drowsiness; therefore, it is best to eat it in the evening. That is why your men fall asleep in the living room after Thanksgiving dinner.

3) If you are on acid suppression medications, see if you can do some work to eliminate your food allergies. This may allow you to reduce the amount of medication or take it less often.

This reduction in acid suppression medication may enhance your absorption of tryptophan. (Caution: Always consult with your health care practitioner prior to altering your medication.)

4) Sex Touching, hugging and sex increases melatonin production. This is one of those natural therapies that is not only good for you, but can be fun. Let's face it; sex is more fun than taking a melatonin pill!

5) Darkness Make sure you turn down your lights, especially after 10 p.m. Millions of you sit all evening with every light in the house on watching TV or using the computer until bedtime. You then turn off the lights and the TV and expect to go to sleep. Remember, your brain takes several hours to make enough melatonin to allow for optimal quality and quantity of sleep. Dim down the lights after 9 or 10 p.m. Try not to watch TV or use the computer after 10 p.m. If you get up at night have a very low intensity night light in the bathroom or use a weak flashlight. Studies have shown, even a quick 1 second flash of light can disrupt melatonin production. If a loved one must read in bed, have them use a book light, that way the remainder of the lights in the bedroom can be turned off. If your bedroom is bright at night, either from security lighting or street lights, buy some black-out curtains. The more light in your bedroom at night the lower your melatonin production.

6) Supplements Melatonin supplements are available at the health store. Millions of Americans over age 40 use them to fall asleep. If you are under age 40, it is best to use melatonin intermittently. The exception to this is people with chronic illnesses. A chronic illness may disrupt your ability to make melatonin; therefore melatonin supplements may be helpful under those circumstances for people younger than 40.

7) Use the lowest dose melatonin supplement that helps you fall asleep. Begin at 1 mg or less sublingual (under the tongue) if possible. You can always increase if you need to. Like any hormone, melatonin works on a feedback mechanism. This means if you take large amounts of supplemental melatonin, it could inhibit your brains production of intrinsic melatonin.

8) Quality We have discussed this several times, I know. But, there is a lot of poor quality melatonin available. If you are going to take a melatonin supplement make sure it has been assayed by the HPLC method to assure purity.

9) Precautions If you have an autoimmune disorder, use melatonin only with the direct supervision of a knowledgeable health care practitioner. Melatonin improves immunity and if you have an autoimmune disorder you may not want to upregulate your immune system further.

10) Your doctor will not be aware of the scientific studies showing melatonins effectiveness. Therefore, consult a health care practitioner that has used and understands melatonins risks and benefits.

Summary

In this chapter we have shown that melatonin can reduce breast cancer risk by as much as 36%. We learned that it does this through its antioxidant effects, ability to improve immunity, and quantity and quality of sleep. You learned that many of you are not able to make normal amounts of melatonin, due to sleep disturbances, nutritional deficiencies or your own bad habits. Improving your level of melatonin is a vital part of your complete breast cancer prevention strategy. Steps you can take to improve your melatonin production are:

1) Increase tryptophan containing foods.

2) Reduce light exposure at night.

3) Turn down the lights to dim in the evenings. Avoid watching late night television or computer.

4) Make sure you are asleep by 1 a.m.

5) If you are on acid suppression mediations, find natural ways to reduce.

6) Sex, touching and hugging all increase melatonin production.

7) If you consider melatonin supplementation, start at a very low dose of a quality melatonin product and increase slowly, in most cases to a maximum of 3 mg per evening. (Most of you will require significantly lower doses to obtain the desired improvements in your sleep.)

8) Avoid melatonin without physician consent if you have lupus, leukemia, lymphoma, rheumatoid arthritis, thyroiditis or any autoimmune disorder.

Let's continue now and review several other natural nutrients that are important for reducing your breast cancer risk by 90% or MORE!

---

[1] Epidemiology (May 1991)
[2] British Journal of Cancer (2001); 84: 397-99.
[3] Conley E. J. America Exhausted; Breakthrough Treatments of Fatigue and Fibromyalgia, Vitality Press (1998)
[4] Journal of the National Cancer Institute (Oct. 2001)
[5] Life Extension Weekly Update (19, Oct. 2001):1-6.

14

More Nutrients That Reduce Your Risk

Lycopene, Lutein and Carotenoids

1) A study in The American Journal of Epidemiology showed women in the lowest 25% for beta-carotene, lutein, and other carotenoids had double the risk of breast cancer as compared to women who were in the highest 25%.[1] DOUBLE THE RISK! Beta-carotene is an antioxidant that is in orange/yellow vegetables. This includes carrots, squash and yams. Lutein is an antioxidant in green leafy vegetables, especially spinach.

2) A Swedish study demonstrated that lutein reduced breast cancer risk in premenopausal women and lycopene reduced the breast cancer risk of postmenopausal women.[2]

These fascinating studies demonstrate that the antioxidants in certain fruits and vegetables reduce your risk of breast cancer by 50%.

What are Antioxidants?

Oxidation is the damage process of nature. Under a variety of circumstances our bodies create "free radicals". These free radicals are electrons and if not neutralized they will slam into DNA and other important cellular structures causing damage. Antioxidants function to absorb these free radicals BEFORE they damage us! The more free radicals you generate, the more antioxidants you require. We generate free radicals through a variety of activities. The process of making energy generates free radicals. We require large amounts of antioxidants every day just to quench the free radicals we generate when we make our energy. Then we do stupid things to generate even more free radicals. Some damage is due to free radical generation from the sun striking our skin or our eyes. Cigarettes damage our tissue through the generation of free radicals, which over the years causes disruption and damage to the DNA of various organs, including the breasts, and eventually results in cancer. Excessive use of alcohol, certain medications and long-term stress all generate large amounts of free radials. The more free radicals we generate, the more antioxidants we use up. If we do not get sufficient antioxidants in our diet, over time we go "bankrupt", i.e. we generate more free radicals than we have antioxidants to quench them. That is when the free radical damage really starts to pile up. Just like a boxer whose arms are down, we start to get pummeled. Eventually more damage is done to our DNA than we can repair. Cells start to reproduce wildly because of this damaged DNA. These wildly reproducing cells eventually become a tumor.

Fruits and vegetables have antioxidants because they need to protect themselves from the sun. Plants must have sunlight to generate energy, yet even for plants this is a double-edged sword since sunlight also can cause free radical damage. That is why your lawn furniture breaks apart in the fall, after it has been outside all summer. The sun has oxidized the furniture through free radical damage, making the furniture more brittle and draining it of its color. Unlike plants and animals, your lawn furniture cannot make antioxidants to protect itself. The color pigments in fruits and vegetables, lutein in spinach, lycopene in tomatoes, carotene in squash or carrots, flavonoids in blueberries or cherries (i.e. the blue in blueberries and the red in cherries) all have been developed by the plant to protect it from sun damage. All animals have developed, over time, an ability to use plant based antioxidants to protect them from free radical damage. We, of course, can make certain antioxidants in our bodies. These include substances like glutathione, which is an important antioxidant we make from three separate amino acids. Other antioxidants, however, we must obtain through the diet. An example would be vitamin C. Humans cannot make vitamin C, we must get it in our diet. The diets of native people contained high amounts of antioxidants since they ate very little processed foods. Most of the foods they ate came directly from nature. The Western diet is very high in processed foods. These foods are very low in antioxidants; therefore, over the years we can develop an antioxidant deficiency. When this antioxidant deficiency is combined with increased oxidative damage, either through cigarettes, alcohol, stress, or normal aging, it creates a dangerous situation where the free radicals are allowed to damage our DNA, causing breaks and/or mutations, which if not repaired eventually can lead to a breast tumor. This is why every study shows that women who eat more fruits and vegetables have a lower risk of breast cancer! Every study I have ever read shows that anyone who eats more fruits and vegetables has a generalized lower risk of all cancers. As we discussed with the beta-carotene/lutein study in The American Journal of Epidemiology, those women in the highest 25% of these two nutrients slashed their breast cancer risk in HALF!

Summary

FIND EASY, DELICIOUS WAYS TO EAT MORE FRUITS AND VEGETABLES! Some simple suggestions would be:

1. Blueberry and/or cherry pie (low sugar added).
2. Carrots, broccoli and cauliflower with dip.

3. Baked winter squash.

4. Great salads with fruits, nuts and mixed greens.

5. Coleslaw.

6. Plums, apples and peaches as snacks.

7. Sautéed summer squash.

8. Tomato soup or sauce.

9. Peppers, broccoli and asparagus in omelets or quiche.

10. Strawberries with whipped cream. (Remember, I said to have fun. A small amount of whipped cream with a bowl of fresh strawberries is a wonderful dessert.)

11. Spinach pie.

12. Melon and cantaloupe in the morning.

13. Herbs: basil, oregano, rosemary, parsley, cilantro in any dish possible.

14. Pumpkin pie (low sugar added).

15. Cool watermelon slices on a hot summer day.

16. Grape juice.

17. Vegetable and/or fruit juice.

These are just a few ideas to show you how much fun eating antioxidants can really be. Look for ways to add fruits and vegetables to all of your meals.

Increasing your antioxidant intake can be delicious, easy and requires little work. Find a grocery or health store that carries organic fruits and vegetables. Remember, this is an integral part of your plan to reduce your risk to breast cancer by at least 90%.

---

[1] Toniolo, The American Journal of Epidemiology
[2] Hulton et al, "Cancer, Causes, and Control" 2001 529-37.

15

Chemicals That Can Cause Breast Cancer

Since the mid 20th Century we have been exposed to thousands of man-made chemicals. We use these chemicals in plastics, pesticides, weed killers, solvents, paints, many other uses. Many of these chemicals resemble or act like an estrogen. (When a chemical has estrogenic properties it is called a xenoestrogen.) We are usually exposed to these chemicals in small doses, but over time they are stored up in our body fat. Over a number of years we can build up significant levels. Since your breasts are 90% fat, they are affected more severely than body organs that contain less fat. These chemicals are stored in breast tissue and bind the estrogen receptors in your breasts. Many of these chemicals irreversibly bind to your estrogen receptors; and stimulate abnormal cellular reproduction. As we have discussed in previous chapters, abnormal cellular reproduction if allowed to continue can eventually cause a tumor. This is how rats are given breast cancer in the laboratory. We give them a chemical like dioxin and we can virtually guarantee that the animals will develop breast cancer. It is not a question of if; it is simply a question of what dose of dioxin will cause their breast cells to become abnormal? We are not talking about high dose exposure, but parts per million and in some cases parts per billion. We know in the laboratory, dioxin causes breast cancer in rats. No one knows what a safe level of dioxin exposure is for you! Greater concern is: what happens when you have exposure to several known carcinogens? The government does not require industry to study the effects of several chemical carcinogens working in unison. Most toxicology studies are conducted using one carcinogen on a lab animal at a time. Independent laboratory studies suggest that these carcinogenic chemicals have a synergistic effect. That means, with exposure to several chemicals it takes less of each (to cause cancer) than if you had a single exposure. If you are thinking that you have not had exposure to these chemicals because you do not work in a factory or industrial setting, you are kidding yourself! We have all been exposed to numerous carcinogens and continue to be exposed every day. It is simply a matter of how much! Studies have shown that dioxin, DDE and PCB have been detected in ice cream, fried chicken, pizza, and hamburgers.[1] This study shows that these chemicals are pervasive in our food. That is because they are everywhere in our environment. Unless you have been locked away in a monastery in Tibet, you have these chemicals in your breasts. Let's review what chemicals are the most dangerous, how to avoid those chemicals, and steps you can take to block these carcinogens from harming YOUR breasts.

What Chemicals are Dangerous?

Unfortunately, there are so many dangerous chemicals in our environment that we could devote a whole book to discussing the chemicals we are exposed to and their dangers. I know it is sad, but true! What we will do in this chapter is give you a primer, so to speak, on the major groups of chemicals that can harm your breasts and how to avoid them.

Dioxin and Dioxin-Like PCBS.

Dioxin is a chemical made from chlorine. It is so toxic that it is measured in trillionths of a gram.[2] Dioxin is used to make plastic wrap, pesticides, wood preservatives, bleached paper and a host of other industrial products. Through these industrial uses dioxin is released into our streams and lakes. It is concentrated in the meat, dairy and fish we eat. In addition, by burning plastic we release dioxins into the air where it may further contaminate soil, water and eventually us. Perhaps the most tragic industrial exposure happened in my home state of Michigan in the 1970's. PCBs were mistakenly placed in cattle feed. The cattle were fed this feed and we then consumed the milk from those cattle. Since that time studies have consistently shown that the majority of women in Michigan have elevated PCBs in their breast milk. Industrial accidents like this are tragic, but as far as we know, fairly rare. A more common problem is that we are exposed to dioxin and dioxin-like chemicals every day through our food.[1] Even more disturbing is that this study done in The European Journal of Cancer found that exposure of an average 6-year-old was especially high "due to a child's lower body weight".[1] (Author's Note: Chemical exposure often produces symptoms in children and pets first. This is due to the fact that they are lower body weight; therefore they do not tolerate as high of an exposure as an adult. One of the subtle questions I always ask my patients is if their children or pets have been sick? Many times after the house has been sprayed with a pesticide the dog or cat will develop leukemia and/or lymphoma. This is a sign that the adults and children have had significant exposure as well.)

A Canadian study of 400 women found a "clear association" with the amount of PCBs measured in breast tissue and breast cancer risk.[3]

Along with dioxin and PCBs, there are several other chemicals that occur in plastics that may be carcinogenic. These include bisphenol-A (a chemical used in plastic milk jugs, bottles, plastic can linings) and phthalates (Used in plastic wrap, deli wrap and plastic bottles).

DDT and DDE

These chemicals have been banned for use in the United States because of their known reproductive toxicity. Yet we allow them to be manufactured in the U.S. and shipped to foreign countries, especially Latin America, where they are sprayed on fruit and vegetables and then imported back to the U.S. (How dumb is that?)

Pesticides

Many pesticides have estrogen-like effects. Organochlorines have been shown to cause breast cancer in lab animals. (DDT is a "banned" organochlorine.) A fascinating study was done on seals that ate herring contaminated with dioxin-like organochlorines in the Baltic. This two year study showed that the seals natural killer cell function was reduced 20-50%.[4] Natural killer cells are responsible for detecting and destroying early cancers. When you reduce natural killer cell function by 20-50%, you are significantly impairing your immune systems response to cancer. This increases the likelihood that a cancer will escape detection and/or destruction and eventually become a tumor. A study published in The Journal of the National Cancer Institute showed breast cancer was 400% higher in the women with the highest levels of organochlorine DDE in their breast tissue.[5] Researchers have found that organochlorines selectively activate the enzyme that converts estrogen to the more dangerous 4 OH and 16 OH metabolites. We have already reviewed that the 4 OH metabolite appears to be a carcinogen.

We have also reviewed that the 16 OH metabolite if elevated increases your risk of breast cancer by reducing your estrogen metabolite index, EMI. For a list of organochlorine pesticides see Table 15A.

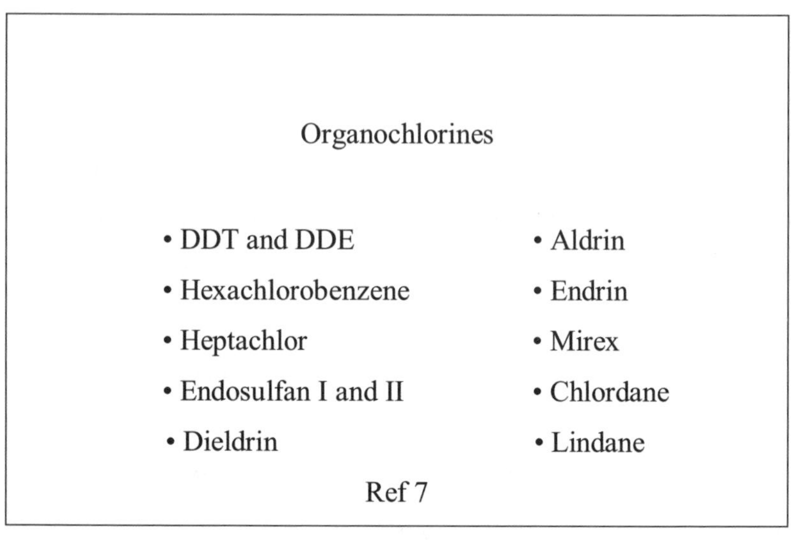

Organochlorines

- DDT and DDE
- Hexachlorobenzene
- Heptachlor
- Endosulfan I and II
- Dieldrin
- Aldrin
- Endrin
- Mirex
- Chlordane
- Lindane

Ref 7

Table 15A

<u>Estrogens in our Meat and Milk</u>

Farmers routinely give estrogen to cattle to make them gain weight more quickly or to help them produce more milk. Since the farmer gets paid by the pound, not the quality, the object is to get cattle fat as quickly as possible. Dairy farmers get paid for their milk by the number of pounds they produce, therefore, you want each cow producing the maximum amount of milk daily. Unfortunately, these hormones go into the meat and milk that you and your family eat every day. Once inside of you guess where these estrogens go? Yes, some of them go to your breasts and attach to your estrogen receptors. This stimulation causes increased cell reproduction. The more meat and milk you eat, the stronger the estrogenic stimulation. Who drinks the most milk, our children! Some scientists have speculated that this is one reason why women are attaining menarche at younger and younger ages. They are getting supplemental estrogen in their food and we just have not recognized it.

What to Do?

Given the dangers presented by these chemicals and the difficulty in avoiding them, what in the world should a reasonable person do? In my opinion the evidence is clear. You should reduce or avoid these chemicals in any way possible! Let's review some simple steps you can take to reduce your chemical exposure and protect yourself and your family.

1) Eat Organic Fruits and Vegetables. Organic fruit and vegetables have not been sprayed with pesticides and/or herbicides. This means they are free of organochlorines and related compounds. These vegetables/fruit are more expensive, but worth every penny. To reduce your costs, you can join an organic food co-op so you can buy in bulk. Even if you wish not to join a co-op, you should find the closest health food store and/or supermarket that have organic produce and purchase your fruits and vegetables there. Not only will your fruits and vegetables be free from pesticides and herbicides, but studies have shown that organic produce is actually HIGHER in vitamins and minerals than non-organically produced produce.[8] Organic milk is also available at health food stores and in an increasing number of traditional supermarkets.
2) Eat Clean Meat/Poultry. Organic meat and poultry can be very expensive to buy. I recommend you buy "clean" meat. What do I mean by clean? Clean meat and poultry have been raised

without estrogen supplementation and with a minimum of chemical exposure. They have not routinely been given antibiotics. By definition this is not organic since organic meat and/or poultry must be fed organic feed. Clean meat/poultry is not perfect, but a darn sight better and safer than commercial meat/poultry. (Author's Note: What I do is buy my meat and poultry directly from farmers that I have interviewed and I know how and what they feed the animals. In this way I am reasonably certain of reducing the amount of pesticides, estrogens and antibiotics I consume in the meat/poultry. I get safer, better tasting meat/poultry at a lower cost than in the supermarket. This is a win-win situation. It takes a little more work in the beginning, but is well worth it.) A good place to start is your local farmer's market. You can interview the local farmers directly and discuss with them how they raise their meat/poultry. Another place would be to contact your local organic food club, since they may know sources in your area of clean and/or reasonably priced organic meat/poultry.

3) Do Not Spray Pesticides and/or Herbicides in Your House, Lawn or Garden. Think before you act! If you have bugs in your house or garden you do not have to live with them. There are plenty of safe, natural, organic ways to get rid of the bugs and/or weeds without getting rid of you or your children. If you needed further proof, studies show that children who live in households where the lawn and garden are routinely sprayed have a 600% higher risk of childhood leukemia than children who live in houses that do not routinely spray. Get rid of the

bugs and/or weeds organically and keep your children and yourself safe.

4) Avoid Plastic Where Possible. This one is tougher. Trying to avoid plastic wraps and bottles where possible. Does anyone remember the milk carton? Trying to avoid plastic wrap, use other types of containers. Never microwave anything in plastic wrap or in a plastic bowl. Use the appropriate microwave-safe glass. Do not store water in plastic jugs or bottles, use glass bottles.

5) Block the Toxic Effects of Dioxin. I3C and DIM have been shown to block the effects of dioxin in breast tissue.[5,6] Dioxin and dioxin-like chemicals use the "Ah" receptor on breast cells. We discussed the "Ah" receptor in Chapter 6 in great detail and the fact that when activated the "Ah" receptor promotes breast cell growth. Dioxin binds to the "Ah" receptor and causes abnormal instructions to go to your DNA; therefore, breast cells reproduce wildly and eventually create a tumor. We know from studies that if I3C and/or DIM are given first, they block the majority of dioxins harmful effects on breast tissue. As we reviewed in Chapter 6, the way I3C and DIM does this is by binding to the "Ah" receptor, and if the "Ah" receptor is occupied by I3C or DIM dioxin cannot attach. In Chapter 6 we discussed the scientific studies that show I3C and/or DIM reduce the cancer causing effects of dioxin (in rats) by as much as 90%.[5] The only problem is that I3C and/or DIM do not bind the "Ah" receptor for long periods of time (unlike dioxin, which may bind irreversibly). Taking moderate amounts of

vegetables and/or supplements containing I3C and/or DIM over a long period of time is more protective than taking a large dose over a shorter period. (Example: Eating 3 pounds of broccoli today and then not eating it again for a year will not get the desired result. It is better for you to eat several servings of cruciferous vegetables per week, every week, as a part of your every day diet.) We have reviewed the controversy regarding supplemental I3C vs DIM. The scientific studies, however, are fairly clear on the fact that DIM protects the "Ah" receptor as well as supplemental I3C. (See Chapter 6 concerning dose and precautions of supplemental DIM/I3C.)

Summary

In my opinion the research is clear concerning dioxin, organochlorines, PCBs, and dioxin-like chemicals: THESE CHEMICALS CAN CAUSE BREAST CANCER! Since we do not know what dose is safe, or indeed if any dose is safe, and suspect that these chemicals act in a synergistic manner, AVOIDANCE is the first and best treatment. You can reduce exposure to these chemicals by:

1. Eat organic fruit/vegetables.
2. Use organic pest and weed solutions.
3. Eat organic milk and milk products.
4. Find clean meat and poultry grown by someone you can interview and trust.
5. Think before you use any solvent, cleaner, spray, degreaser or paint in your house or your life. Read all labels carefully. Use natural and organic alternatives that are available at larger health stores.

6. Eat cruciferous vegetables every day or several times per week. (Caution: Avoid cruciferous vegetables if pregnant or breast feeding.)

7. Consider DIM supplementation if you cannot or will not eat cruciferous vegetables on a regular basis. (See Chapter 6.)

This information is meant as an "eye-opener", not as an exhaustive review of the dangers presented by xenoestrogen chemicals. YOU ALONE are responsible for the health of you and your family. You must know what you are eating, how it is grown and where it came from. You should know what chemicals are used and/or sprayed in your house, garden and lawn, as they can pose a significant cancer risk to your family. (Do not take the manufacturers word on this. In addition, pesticides and/or lawn companies will rarely be up front on the possible dangers involved. Therefore, buyer beware.) In short, you can, with very little work, avoid many exposures to these chemicals and improve the quality of your life in the process. Unfortunately, all of us will continue to get exposure to dioxin and other organochlorines every time we eat out. For these exposures you can help block the harmful effects by eating cruciferous vegetables several times per week and/or taking an I3C or DIM supplement. Include in your daily diet as many organic fruits and vegetables as possible, since the antioxidants included in these foods will help reduce your risk of breast cancer.

Avoidance of chemicals is another dramatic step you can take to reduce your risk of breast cancer by 90% or more.

---

[1] Schecter A et al., "Dioxins, Dibenzofurans, Dioxin-like PCBs, and DDE in U.S. Fast Food," (1995) Chemosphere, Volume 34 #5-7:1449-57, 1997 (European Journal of Cancer)

[2] "Beat the Odds against Breast Cancer," Great Life Magazine (October 2001):32-35.
[3] Colburn T et al., "Our Stolen Future," Publisher Dutton/Signet Books (1996)
[4] Wolff M S et al., "Blood Levels of Organochlorine Residue and Risk of Breast Cancer," The Journal of National Cancer Institute 85 (8) (1993):468-652.
[5] Bradlow et al., "13C: A Novel Approach to Breast Cancer Prevention," Annals of New York Academy of Science (1995); 76:180-200.
[6] Chen I et al., "13C and DIM as Aryl Hydrocarbon (Ah) Receptor Agonists and Antagonists in T47D Human Breast Cancer Cells," Biochem Pharma, Vol. 51: 1069-76 (1996)
[7] William J Rea, M.D. "Chemical Sensitivity, Vol. IV:2106
[8] Smith B L "Organic Foods vs Supermarket Foods: Element Levels" Journal of Applied Nutrition, Vol 45: No 1 (1993)

16

Low B12 and Folate Increase Breast Cancer Risk

A study published in 1999 showed that low B12 appears to be a risk factor for breast cancer. That study found that there was an increased risk of breast cancer in the 20% of postmenopausal women who had the lowest B12 levels as compared with the other 80% with higher levels. [1] B12 deficiency could increase your risk for breast cancer through at least three different mechanisms:

1) Low B12 may contribute to producing what is known as a folate trap. We need a type of folate named 5, 10-methylene tetrahydrofolate to make something named thymidine. Thymidine is important in making and repairing DNA. We require B12 to convert folate to this 5, 10-methylene tetrahydrofolate. If you are low in B12, you cannot make this conversion and since 5, 10 methylene tetrahydrofolate is required to make thymidine, you may run low in thymidine. Here is where it gets interesting. If your body runs low in thymidine, it may insert another nucleotide named Uracil into your DNA in place of thymidine. Your body, however, knows this is a mistake and removes the Uracil and by doing so causes one strand of your DNA to break. We have already talked about the fact that DNA is double-stranded, meaning, there are two distinct copies. The problems start when you get this single strand break in both copies of your DNA. This can eventually lead to a mutation in that gene. We have already talked about the fact that breast cancer starts with genetic damage and mutation. Therefore, if this double-strand break happens in your breast tissue, you will get a genetic mutation in your breast cells which could cause cancer.

2) Your tumor suppressor genes require methylation in order to function. The lower the methylation, the greater reduction in function of tumor suppressor genes. Two substances that are very important in methylation are B12 and folate. Each of these substances contributes methyl groups to various processes in the body improving function. In this case, they would contribute methyl groups to your tumor suppressor genes, therefore, up regulating those genes. We have already discussed the fact you want your tumor suppressor genes upregulated (more active) not down regulated. Studies have shown that DNA in breast cancer had significantly lower methylation compared with normal breast tissue. [2]

3) Studies have shown that increased methylation of tumor promoter genes turn those genes off, which reduces breast cancer risk. [3] So, not only does increased methylation improve tumor suppressor genes, but it also reduces tumor promoter genes. You want your tumor suppressor genes to be turned up and your tumor promoter genes to be turned down. These studies suggest B12 and folate, since they are excellent methyl group donors, help turn up your tumor suppressor genes and turn down your tumor promoter genes.

An interesting study was done as part of the Iowa Women's Health Study. This study of 4,000 women age 55-69 concluded that as long as women who drank alcohol had enough folate they were not at an increased risk of breast cancer. It showed that women who drank 4 grams of alcohol a day, but had the highest folate levels were at no greater risk of breast cancer than a woman who did not drink. However, women who drank only two grams of alcohol per day, but were in the lowest 25% of folate had a 59% higher risk of breast cancer.[4] We know that the detoxification of alcohol depletes folate. Therefore, the more alcohol you drink the more folate you need. It is unfortunate that the vast majority of American women are already low in folate. That is why it is now recommended that pregnant women take at least 400 mcg of folate daily. Folate (folic acid) has been shown to reduce neuro tube defects in newborns.

How Do You Know if You are Low in B12 and Folate?

There are two ways.

1) Since most American women are deficient in both, supplementation of both makes sense. We will discuss this shortly.

2) You can have your levels measured. If you go to your family doctor and ask for B12 and folate levels, he/she will do a serum B12 and folate level. If they are low or low normal, you know you need B12 and folate supplementation. If they are "within normal range" that does not necessarily mean you have enough B12/folate. The reason for this is that serum B12/folate levels have such a wide range of normal. You can be within "normal range" and still not have enough folate/B12 to turn up your tumor suppressor genes and turn down your tumor promoter genes. To fully evaluate your B12 and folate levels, your doctor should do homocystine, methylmalonate and tetrahydrofolate levels. These levels more accurately reflect your true B12/folate status. B12 and folate are required to convert homocystine to the amino acid methionine. If you are low in B12 and folate, you will not make this conversion and homocystine levels will go up. Elevated homocystine is a risk factor for heart disease and cancer, since it indicates that you are functionally low in B12 and folate. Elevated methylmalonate levels suggest a functional B12 deficiency, since B12 is required for the conversion of methylmalonate. Tetrahydrofolate is the type of folate that is active in the body. One out of every five Americans has trouble converting folate to tetrahydrofolate. (If your tetrahydrofolate levels are low, you may require a tetrahydrofolate supplement or much higher doses of folic acid.)

What Can You Do if your B12 and Folate Levels are Low?

Diet

Dietary sources of folate are green leafy vegetables, peas, beans and enriched cereals. Sources of B12 are meats including liver, fish, beef, and fortified cereals. (Three ounces of liver contains 60 mcg of B12. Three ounces of beef contains 2.1 mcg. Three ounces of salmon/trout contains approximately 5 mcg.) Most Americans no longer eat liver. Unless the liver was from an organic cow, it is probably not worth eating.

<u>Supplements</u>

B12 and folate are very easily and inexpensively supplemented. There are essentially no known side effects to reasonable doses of either. Since folate deficiency is widespread throughout the American population, supplementation with 400 mcg to 1 mg per day makes sense. B12 can be supplemented at approximately 1000 mcg daily sublingual (under the tongue). My preferred type of B12 supplement is methylcobalamin. The more common form of B12 supplement is cyanocobalamin, which is B12 combined with small amounts of cyanide. While these small amounts of cyanide have never been shown to have any deleterious effects, it makes sense to me to use the methylcobalamin form since we are trying to increase the amounts of methyl groups available within the body. (For review of the B12 and folate used in my office, please see the products chapter in the back of this book.) If you use alcohol in moderation it makes sense to supplement B12 and folate. The dose I use in the office is 400 mcg to 1 mg daily. For my patients that drink alcohol frequently, I often recommend a higher dose of folate (1-3 mg daily) and B12 (1000-3000 mcg daily). As we have discussed, those women who drank alcohol, but were in the lowest 20% of folate intake, had a <u>60% higher</u> risk of breast cancer.

The moral of this story is, do not allow B12 and folate deficiency to increase your risk of breast cancer! Folate and B12 supplementation is cheap, easy, and if done in moderation essentially free of side effects. There is really no reason why you should allow B12 and folate deficiency to increase your risk of breast cancer.

Now lets move on to see how improving the "ninjas" of your immune system can help to reduce your breast cancer risk by 90% or more.

---

[1] Wu "A Prospective Study on Folate, B12, and Pyridoxal 5-phosphate (B6) and Breast Cancer," Cancer Epidemiol Biomarkers Prevention (1999); 8: 209-17.

[2] Soares J. Pinto, AE, Cunha CB et al., "Global DNA Hypomethylation in Breast Carcinoma"Journalist Cancer (1999); 85: 112-118.

[3] Nutritional Reviews, Vol. 57, 8" 250-3 "Vitamin B12 Deficiency: A New Risk Factor for Breast Cancer?"

[4] Author Unknown, Eurekalert Press Release Associated Press, "Folate Acid, Breast Cancer and Alcohol Consumption Life Extension" (Aug 2001): p 16

17

Improve Your Cancer Fighting Immune Cells

The most important step you can take to improve your immunity is to improve your natural killer cell function. (NK function)

What are NK cells?

Natural killer cells (NK) are the "special forces" of the immune system. Like military special forces, they are small in numbers, but very important in the "seek and destroy" mission of the immune system. NK cells are responsible for recognizing intruders, attacking those intruders and destroying them. When NK cells attack, they produce chemicals that stimulate the remainder of your immune system to move to the area of the body that is infected. This is important for defense from viruses, bacteria, parasites, and CANCER. NK cells are responsible for detecting the 200 cancers each of us develop every day. Of the trillions of cells in our body, millions become sick, damaged or mutated daily. The majority of these sick cells self-destruct in a process we call apoptosis. Cancer cells lose this ability to self-destruct. Therefore, several hundred cancers may begin each and every day. It is the job of NK cells to recognize these deformed, mutated cells (i.e. cancer) and destroy them.

There are two important factors in determining NK cell effectiveness. 1. The number of NK cells. 2. The function of those cells. Like the military Special Forces you can have two problems. 1) Not enough soldiers. 2) Enough soldiers, but they do not fight very well. Of these two problems, the most dangerous is soldiers that do not fight well, in other words, NK cells that do not function well. AIDS research has shown that a person can be surprisingly healthy with very few NK cells as long as normal function is maintained. If a person with AIDS loses NK cell function, even if their numbers are near normal, they develop cancers such as sarcoma and die. In this chapter we will focus on how to improve your NK cell function so your body can easily detect and kill breast cancer BEFORE these cancers endanger your life.

How Do YOU Know Your NK Cell Function Level?

Anyone can have their NK cell function measured. A blood sample is taken and the NK cells that are removed (within 24 hours) are subjected to stimuli to see how well they attack. In the right laboratory this is easily done. (Author's Note: This NK cell function, however, is not a routine test and one that most doctors and/or laboratories may not be familiar with. This study requires a special laboratory.) Measurement of your NK cell function is actually fairly easy as long as you have a doctor and laboratory familiar with the procedure.

What Lowers Natural Killer Cell Function?

No one is absolutely sure of all the factors that reduce NK cell function. One can point to some of the usual suspects: Stress, poor diet, nutritional deficiency, lack of sleep, viral infection and depression. Significant research has been done on NK cell function in AIDS, but very little research has been done on the factors that depress NK cells in a less sick population.

If your NK Cell Function is Low, What Can be Done to Improve It?

Research has shown several supplements which improve NK cell function. Before we discuss these, let's make sure that you have covered some of the basics.

1) Increase your sleep. See Melatonin Chapter 13.

2) Reduce stress.

3) Improve your diet.

4) Reduce or regulate depression: Keep blood sugars stable and use nutrients to maintain normal brain chemistry. (For discussion of the many nutrients that help fight depression, sign up for the free monthly newsletter "Vitality Today". In this newsletter, I discuss many of the nutrients important to mental health and physical energy. These nutrients include SAMe, Tryptophan, St. John's Wort, Tyrosine, etc. To find out how to subscribe, see the product/services section at the back of this book.)

Supplements

- Glutathione (GTH). This is a 3 amino acid antioxidant that is vital for detoxification and cellular protection. Studies have shown glutathione improves natural killer cell function.

How Do You Know if You are Low in Glutathione?

There are several laboratory studies available that measure glutathione levels. If you are over 40 and have been on the Standard America Diet (SAD), odds are you are deficient in this important nutrient. This deficiency is compounded by alcohol use (the liver requires GTH to detoxify alcohol), toxins, smoking and medications. GTH is a very important antioxidant in the detoxification of estrogen. Remember, all estrogen is detoxified in the liver to its metabolites. If you are low in GTH your detoxification slows down.

How Do you Improve your GTH Levels?

1) NAC (N-acetyl cysteine): This is an amino acid that is important in the production of glutathione and is well absorbed when given orally.

2) Glutamine: Another amino acid that is important for glutathione production within the body.

3) GTH: Glutathione does come as a supplement, but is more poorly absorbed than NAC. If you use GTH as a supplement, make sure it is in reduced form, since only reduced glutathione functions as an antioxidant. (Caution: Diabetics should not take GTH supplements without the expressed consent of their physicians since GTH may alter their blood sugars.)

4) Lipoic acid: This is an antioxidant that helps recharge glutathione into the reduced form. When glutathione soaks up a free radical it is then oxidized. Lipoic acid absorbs the free radical from glutathione converting it back into the reduced form, which is the form that can function as an antioxidant.

I cannot stress enough the point that quality supplements make all the difference in the world. There are "tricks" manufacturers use to reduce the price of supplements for example, if you buy glutathione that is not in reduced form you are wasting your money! For further information on the supplements I recommend, please see the product section at the end of the book.

IP-6 (Inositol hexaphosphate)

1) IP-6 is the nutrient that results when 6 phosphate groups are attached to the B vitamin Inositol.

2) Cereals and legumes are the richest natural sources of IP-6.

3) IP-6 helps prevent breast cancer by controlling the rate of cellular division. Studies have shown IP-6 was effective in inhibiting both estrogen receptor positive and estrogen receptor negative breast cell lines.

4) IP-6 also improves natural killer cell function. Studies have shown that IP-6 can upregulate the function of your natural killer cells.

5) Dose. The usual dose of IP-6 is two capsules twice daily.

6) Side effects. Few side effects have been observed with IP-6 since it is simply a B vitamin attached to six groups of phosphate.

7) Caution: You should not use IP-6 if you have an autoimmune disorder.

Discussion

Clinically I have used IP-6 on hundreds of patients who were found to have low NK cell function. Combining natural therapies with replacement of nutritional deficiencies, in conjunction with IP-6 has allowed many of those patients to regain more normal NK cell function. Improved NK cell function enables them to fight off infection and cancer.

MGN-3

MGN-3 is a nutrient that is originally derived from mushrooms. Studies have shown that 3000 mg of MGN-3 per day increased the activity of NK cells by as much as 300%.1[1]

Summary

I recommend that you know what your natural killer cell function level is. If it is low, take steps to improve it. These steps include:

1) Increasing and improving your sleep.

2) Reducing stress.

3) Improving your diet.

4) Improving or resolving depression.

5) If after 3-6 months, your NK cell function has not improved upon recheck, then the addition of supplements, including glutathione, lipoic acid, IP-6 and/or MGN-3 should be considered. (Caution: Do not take MGN-3 if you are allergic to mushrooms.)

By improving your NK cell function, you increase the likelihood that your body's immune system will detect and destroy early breast cancers. Most doctors do not directly work with natural killer cell function, therefore, they will not be familiar with the research and/or how to measure it. To have your NK cell function measured see the product/services section at the back of this book. Prior to implementing any supplement program, make sure you consult a physician who understands nutritional therapy.

---

[1] Ghoneum Mamdooh, PhD, Townsend Letter for Doctors and Patients. (January 2000)

18

Detoxify to Reduce Your Breast Cancer Risk

We have discussed that estrogen is detoxified in the liver to its metabolites via the P-450 pathway. Significant amounts of these estrogen metabolites go back into your circulation. To maintain balance, your body must be able to get rid of excessive estrogen and estrogen metabolites. It does this through a detoxification pathway named Glucuronidation. Once estrogen is detoxified via this Glucuronidation pathway, it is excreted in the stool and urine. If you are unable to get rid of these metabolites, they are reabsorbed from the bowel and reenter your circulation. Millions of women have the complaint of chronic constipation. Many women have a movement every 3-7 days and think that it is "normal." Yet, the longer you allow these estrogen metabolites to stay in the body, the more they will be reabsorbed and reenter circulation. This, of course, increases the levels of estrogen metabolites in your blood. We have already discussed that the lower your levels of the "bad" 16 OH and 4 OH metabolites, the better. Once these metabolites are excreted into your bowel, the key is to eliminate them so they are not reabsorbed.

Constipation

It is hard for many women to realize how constipation can be so damaging to their health and how your bowel can possibly affect your breasts. The Ancient Chinese put it bluntly when they said, "Death begins in the bowel." Millions of American women have chronic constipation because their bowel is "sick". If your bowel is sick, you cannot absorb the nutrients necessary for health, your immunity suffers, and your energy plummets. A sick bowel has an overgrowth of "bad bacteria". These "bad bacteria" produce an enzyme named beta-glucuronidase. Normal substances like hormones and harmful chemicals like pesticides are bound to glucarate in the liver and removed via our stool. If the harmful enzyme beta-glucuronidase is high, toxins and hormones cannot bind to glucarate and are kept in our body. This increases both the levels of free estrogen and levels of estrogen metabolites. Elevated levels of free estrogen and/or beta-glucuronidase are associated with increase risk of breast cancer. [1-2] A sick bowel also loses its peristalsis. (Author's Note: Peristalsis is the normal muscular contraction of the bowel that keeps waste products moving.) A reduction of peristalsis causes hormones and toxins to stay in the bowel for longer periods of time. As we discussed before, many of them get reabsorbed.

<u>Why Do Millions of Women have a "Sick Bowel?</u>

There are many ways your bowel can become "sick". The most common reason in Western societies is <u>overuse of antibiotics.</u> Baby-boomers and every generation since have grown up with antibiotics both as prescriptions and in our food. Most of us have had many courses of prescription antibiotics by the time we are adults. Those of you with allergies or chronic ear/throat problems had multiple courses of antibiotics during your childhood. Some of you, as teens, had years of antibiotics for acne. Then with sexual activity you had urinary tract infections and vaginal infections all requiring even more antibiotics. What you have not been told is that every time you take an antibiotic it not only kills the "bad" bacteria that we are trying to kill, but it kills the "good" bacteria that are vital for digestion. (Author's Note: You know that the first thing that happens when you take an antibiotic is you get a vaginal yeast infection. The reason for this is the antibiotic kills off the "good" bacteria that helps protect your vagina, but does not kill yeast. This allows the yeast to overgrow and causes an infection.) After many courses of antibiotics, the good bacteria in your bowel becomes decimated. Since your bowel is absolutely dependent on good bacteria for normal function it starts to become "sick." As the good bacteria are killed bad bacteria or yeast, which are resistant to antibiotics overgrow, thereby reducing the absorption of nutrients from your food and producing toxins, which cause a number of adverse health affects. Good bacteria produce nutrients that are necessary to feed the inner lining of your digestive tract. (This is one of the few places in the body where nutrients are not received directly from the blood.) As the good bacteria become decimated, they produce fewer nutrients. As the nutrient levels drop, your bowel cannot get the proper nourishment and starts to become more damaged leading to the point where function becomes seriously impaired. Doctors have been ignorant of this problem; therefore they have never told you to replace the good bacteria to maintain proper bowel health. Good bacteria can be replaced by eating foods that are high in good bacteria like yogurt, buttermilk or kefir or by taking probiotics (good bacteria supplements). There are literally dozens of studies that show post-antibiotic super infections are dramatically reduced with probiotic supplementation. Many of you have had a sick bowel for years, possibly decades. If your bowel is sick, you cannot be healthy. If you do not actively repair the damage that has been done to your bowel, you will be sick for the rest of your life. Repairing a sick bowel is not always easy, but you can start by eating some organic yogurt every day or taking a live probiotic supplement. Some of you will need to have treatment for the overgrowth of yeast or pathogenic bad bacteria along with supplementation of good bacteria. Ninety-million Americans complain of bowel problems, with approximately forty-five million having IRRITABLE BOWEL SYNDROME (IBS). Millions of you have been told by your doctor that IBS is in your head, but in reality it results, in many cases, from destruction of good bacteria and the overgrowth of bad bacteria and/or yeast.

There are other contributing factors to chronic constipation. This includes the lack of fiber: The Standard American Diet (SAD) contains less fiber than any diet in human history. We need fiber to make our bowel function properly.

<u>Water</u>

Many of you drink caffeinated drinks like coffee or soda which further dehydrate. Proper amounts of water are necessary for normal digestion and bowel function.

<u>Exercise</u>

Americans get less exercise than any civilization in human history. Exercise is vital for stimulating the bowel and contributing to normal movements.

<u>Thyroid</u>

Millions of you have subtle low thyroid (hypothyroid). You are cold all the time. You gain weight easily. You are chronically constipated. Many of you have had blood tests that said you were "normal". A new study in <u>The British Medical Journal</u> suggests that our definition of "normal" is incorrect. Usually thyroid stimulating hormone (TSH) has been considered normal if they were between 0.4 and 5.5. (Author's Note: TSH is a hormone produced by our brain that tells our thyroid we need more thyroid hormone. Therefore, TSH goes up when we are thyroid deficient.) This new study states that "normal" TSH should be between 1 and 2, not 5.5. This means many of you were told your thyroid was normal, when in fact you had mild hypothyroidism. If you are cold all of the time, gain weight easily, have dry skin and chronic constipation have your thyroid levels rechecked. If your TSH is above 2, consider low dose thyroid supplementation. An even better test is a 24-hour urine evaluation of thyroid function. This detects subtle low thyroid that blood levels can miss. For further information, see products/services section at the back of this book.

Summary

1. You cannot be healthy if your bowel is sick.

2. Chronic constipation increases the reabsorption of estrogen and estrogen metabolites, thereby INCREASING your risk of breast cancer.

3. The abnormal "bad bacteria" in a sick bowel produces the enzyme beta-glucuronidase, which reduces detoxification of estrogen and INCREASES your risk of breast cancer.

4. A sick bowel cannot absorb the nutrients and antioxidants necessary for health. Therefore, your immunity drops, which INCREASES your risk of breast cancer.

5. Millions of you have developed a "sick bowel" through the overuse of antibiotics, which has killed your good bacteria. To repair the bowel, you must actively replace normal bacteria through foods, supplements or both. (For the good bacteria supplement I recommend, see the product section at the back of this book). Remember, the bacteria must be alive and able to survive your stomach acid.

6. If your bowel is overgrown with yeast and/or "bad bacteria", you must have the correct therapy to reduce the concentration of both of these pathogens. I recommend a complete digestive stool analysis (CDSA) to determine your levels of abnormal bacteria and/or yeast. Regular stool tests done at a traditional laboratory do not check for yeast and pathogenic "bad bacteria". (See products section)

7. Increase your fiber, water and walking to help improve chronic constipation.

8. If you complain of being cold when others are not, you gain weight easily, your skin is dry and you have chronic constipation have your thyroid levels checked. If your 24-hour urine thyroid levels are low or TSH high thyroid supplementation should be considered.

9. As the Ancient Chinese said, "Death begins in the bowel." To reduce your risk of breast cancer by 90% or more you must actively work to restore bowel health.

---

[1] Life Extension (Nov 2000): p 20

[2] Dwivedi C; et al., "Effect of Calcium Glucarate on B-Glucurmidase Activity and Glucarate Content of Certain Vegetables and Fruits" Biochemical Medicine and Metabolic Biology 43: 83-92 (1990)

19

Easy Diet Tips to Reduce Risk

At my book signings throughout the country, I have found that most women, deep down, KNOW that increasing the fruits and vegetables in their diet will reduce their risk of breast cancer. The sad thing is, even though they know this in their heart, they don't do it. The most common reason they give is that they are "too busy". In this chapter, we will not only summarize the foods that help you prevent breast cancer, but also give you easy tips to incorporate these changes into your everyday diet. Let's face it, if the diet is too strict or too hard to follow, you won't do it for very long. We will try to make this simple! Investment advisors always tell you, put whatever amount of money you can into your retirement account, if you can fully fund it every year, terrific! If you cannot then at least put whatever you can afford into your retirement account and make it a yearly habit. This is an excellent analogy for your diet to prevent breast cancer. My hope would be that you can eat five servings a day of fruits and vegetables, but if you cannot or will not, eat as many servings as you can. A very large study called the Nurses Health Study found that premenopausal women who ate five or more servings of fruits and vegetables per day had a lower risk of breast cancer than those who ate fewer than two servings.[1] If eating five servings a day significantly lowers your breast cancer risk, why don't you do it? Women gave several reasons:

1) Not enough time. For some reason, people think that preparation of fruits and vegetables takes time. In reality, nothing can be simpler. How difficult is it to pre-wash some vegetables, for example: broccoli, carrots, snow peas, (you can put in whatever vegetables you like) and use them as a snack throughout the day with some nice, tasty, low-fat, organic ranch dressing as a dip. It is great tasting and fabulous for your health. We have already discussed how important the cruciferous vegetables are to converting your estrogen to the "good" 2 OH metabolite. Using broccoli and cauliflower as a snack is a great way to increase your cruciferous vegetable intake. Have a peach with breakfast, an apple as a snack, strawberries with cream or a small amount of whipped cream for dessert or even a piece of low-sugar blueberry pie. All of these are delicious, easy ways to get more antioxidants in your diet.

2) Vegetables are boring. Vegetables are only boring if you allow them to be. Have fun with your food and make sure it is delicious. There are many easy recipes available that show you how to make vegetables. A common misconception is that to be healthy, you must eat your vegetables plain. I will make a deal with you. I will not force you to eat plain vegetables and I will show you ways to make them delicious if you promise me you will eat more of them. Coleslaw is a great way to increase cabbage in your diet. Yes, I know coleslaw has a small amount of sugar. Keep the amount of sugar as low as possible and use a lower fat, organic coleslaw dressing. Salads. You can buy pre-made gourmet organic salad mixes already prepared at the health store. Use organic tomatoes, broccoli spears, a small amount of fresh fruit (such as tangerines slices) and a few walnuts. Top this off with low-fat organic salad dressing and you have a tremendous food for prevention of breast cancer. Wasn't that easy? You can make this salad twice per week. You do not have to make it daily. Salads will keep for 2-3 days in an appropriate container in the refrigerator. So instead of having a candy bar, a cigarette or soda during your break, have a piece of fruit. It is delicious, high energy and contains antioxidants/fiber/vitamins & minerals. Have a piece of fresh fruit daily for breakfast. Slice up a large bowl of fruit and keep it in the refrigerator. Last, have sliced fruit and/or fruit pie for

dessert. Sliced strawberries with cream or a small amount of whipped cream are a wonderful way to end a meal. If you choose to have pumpkin/blueberry/cherry pie, make sure it is homemade, organic fruit and low sugar. Many commercial pies are basically artificial fruit filling that do not contain antioxidants, are very high in sugar and are worthless.

Brainwashing

Most of us have been raised at a time when we were bombarded by billions of dollars of advertising, conditioning us to buy foods that if consumed on a regular basis will kill us. When we were children, we saw thousands of commercials for sugar coated cereals, fast foods, candy bars and more. The result of all this conditioning is that we spend money to eat foods that are harmful to our health. (For the record, I want to state that there is not a great problem with having a burger and fries or a high sugar dessert occasionally, if done in moderation, these can be a fun "sin"). The problem is that for many of you, these have become staples of your diet. Like alcohol, a small amount now and then can be one of life's little pleasures.

Always Use Organic Fruits and Vegetables

In the chapter on chemicals we discussed how pesticides helped promote breast cancer development. We reviewed that you cannot wash these pesticides off and that once consumed the pesticides will stay with you for life. Even worse, most pesticides are stored in fat; therefore the concentrations in your breasts will be thirty to one thousand times higher than the concentrations in your blood. One good rule to follow for fruits and vegetables is: EAT ORGANIC.

Summary

Eat as many servings of fruit and vegetables per day as possible. Make sure those fruits and vegetables are organic. Here are some easy, fun ways to add fruit/vegetables to your diet.

1) Tomato soup. A warm bowl of tomato soup on a cold winter's day is a great way to get antioxidants. Tomato sauce is another way of getting the power of lycopene in your diet.

2) Chili/vegetable soup. Chili and/or vegetable soup are terrific in the winter and a great way to increase your vegetable intake. Add as many vegetables as possible to the soup. Use organic chicken or beef stock.

3) Vegetable Juice. If you have a juicer at home (I recommend one), you can make your own fresh squeezed vegetable and fruit juices.

4) Snacks. Have carrots, broccoli, cauliflower, and celery sticks prepared and available as snacks. Use a low-fat ranch dressing as dip.

5) Salads. Make "real" salads out of mixed greens with tomatoes, broccoli, zucchini, fruit and nuts. Find a healthy salad dressing you enjoy.

6) Coleslaw or sauerkraut. These are two great ways to increase cabbage in your diet.

7) Fruit. Fresh apple, peach, plum or orange in the morning or as snacks. Sliced or whole berries with or without cream for dessert. Blueberry, strawberry or cherry pie (low sugar added) as dessert.

Change your Oil. No, I am not talking about your car's oil. You are eating too much fat and especially the wrong type of fat. Most of the oil that is in the Standard American Diet (SAD) is omega 6 fatty acids. The omega 6 fatty acids include corn, soy, cottonseed, safflower and peanut oil. Most baked goods and fried foods in the United States contain these types of oil. Margarine is made from omega 6 fatty acids that have been "tortured". What I mean by tortured is, oil does not stay solid at room temperature, it is a liquid. To keep margarine solid at room temperature they torture the oil via a process named hydrogenation. Hydrogenated oils are being linked to a host of health problems, including an increased risk of breast cancer. Researchers found that those women who ate the most polyunsaturated fat had a 69% increased risk of breast cancer.[2] Originally these hydrogenated oils were thought to be better for you than saturated fat. That is why all of our mothers were told to switch to margarine from butter. Another reason for hydrogenated oils popularity is they do not smoke at high temperatures. Therefore they are perfect for fried foods like French fries. We now know these hydrogenated oils increase cardiac risk, not decrease it, and have been shown to increase the risk of breast cancer. I have two rules. Rule 1) Never eat anything that does not spoil easily. Rule 2) Never eat anything that wild animals will not eat. (Just leave a tub of margarine out in your back yard and see if anything will eat it. Even skunks and ants will not touch it.

What Type of Oil Should You Substitute for the Omega-6 Hydrogenated Oils?

Omega-3

These are the oils in ocean fish, flaxseed and other seeds and nuts, including canola. We have already discussed how beneficial flaxseeds and flax oil are in preventing breast cancer. If you are cooking at high temperatures i.e. sautéing or frying, then canola oil is the choice since it does not smoke at high temperature. Any other oil should be olive oil. Olive oil is technically an omega 9 fatty acid, but it has been shown to have many healthy benefits associated with it. Societies that use olive oil have lower risk of heart disease and cancer than Americans. In addition, olive oil has been used with health benefits for over eight thousand years and it tastes great! Make sure you use organic, cold pressed virgin olive oil.

Low Sugar

Sugar intake has been linked with breast cancer in postmenopausal women.[3] You should keep your diet as low in refined sugar as possible. The best way to do this is by reducing your junk food. Commercially available pies, cakes and candies all contain, predominantly sugar. As we discussed before, many commercially available blueberry pies have very few blueberries and are mostly blue sugar syrup. You get the sugar without the antioxidants. (That is a pretty lousy deal!) Get the majority of your sugar through fruit and fruit juices. (Caution: If you have diabetes or hypoglycemia, you will not be able to eat as many servings of fruit or fruit juice as a "normal" person. You can compensate for this by eating more vegetables and/or taking an antioxidant supplement.)

Soy

We have already discussed how beneficial soy can be for improving the detoxification of estrogen (i.e. raising the 2 OH metabolite levels and decreasing 16 OH).

Cruciferous Vegetables

We have also discussed how brussel sprouts, broccoli, kale, cabbage, turnips, collards and cauliflower improve your EMI (2 OH ÷ 16 OH ratio).[4] Increase your cruciferous vegetable intake in every way possible. (Caution: Avoid cruciferous vegetables if you are pregnant or breast-feeding.)

Antioxidants

We have reviewed how green tea and curcumin can slow the growth of breast cancer by inhibiting cell growth at two separate stages named G1 and G2. Additionally, other spices including rosemary can enhance the metabolism of estrogen.[5] Therefore, including rosemary in as many dishes as possible can be helpful.

Yogurt

We have reviewed how eating organic yogurt can help replace the normal bacteria in your bowel, thereby improving bowel function, reducing constipation and allowing for better elimination of estrogen metabolites.

All of these dietary recommendations are so easy and so delicious. It would be a shame for you not to institute them. I hope you see how simple this can be. It does not have to be time consuming. Vegetables and fruit do not have to be boring. We make them so. There are delicious recipes available. Find the recipes that you enjoy and that taste good to you and utilize them.

Lastly, deprogram yourselves from the commercials on television. Remember, those commercials are there to sell a product and to make money. They are not there for the public interest or benefit. They are not designed to keep you from getting breast cancer. Throughout the course of this book we have discussed various nutritional supplements that can help improve your estrogen metabolism and reduce your risk of breast cancer. There are, however, nutrients in foods that we still have not discovered. The majority of your antioxidants and nutrients should come from your food. The addition of supplements will then allow you to bolster your antioxidant/nutrient intake and these two steps (your improved diet and selected antioxidant/nutritional supplements) are a dynamic 1-2 punch in helping you to reduce your risk of breast cancer by 90% or more.

---

[1] Lancet (18, May 1996);347:1351-56
[2] Archives of Internal Medicine (12, January 1998)
[3] Great Life Magazine (October 2001):33-35
[4] Fowke J H et al. "Brassica Vegetable Consumption Shifts Estrogen Metabolism In Healthy Postmenopausal Women" Journal Cancer Epidemiol Biomarkers Prevention (August 2000);9:773-779
[5] Carcinogenesis, Volume 19 #10 (1998):1821-27

20

A Brief Word About SERMS

SERMS are the only treatment traditional medicine has available to reduce your breast cancer risk. The other treatment is to remove both breasts. This is the most radical possible treatment and one that most women would find unacceptable. SERM stands for selective estrogen receptor modulators. These are prescription medications that can act like either an estrogen or an anti-estrogen, dependent on how they are designed and the tissue to which they are exposed. The two most common SERMS are Raloxifene (Evista ™) and Tamoxifen (Nolvadex™).

Raloxifene

Advantages:

- Approved for the treatment of osteoporosis.
- Reduces breast cancer risk. (Not yet approved by the FDA.)
- Does not appear to increase the risk of uterine cancer. (See Tamoxifen.)

Disadvantages:

- Does not reduce menopausal symptoms including hot flashes, night sweats, sleep disturbances, and/or cognitive dysfunction. May actually increase hot flashes.
- Increases the risk of venous thrombosis. (Blood clots of the veins.)

Tamoxifen

Advantages:

- Approved for breast cancer prevention in high risk women only.
- Approved for the treatment of breast cancer or metastatic breast cancer.

Disadvantages:

- Black box warning of serious and life-threatening events with the use of Tamoxifen including increased risk of:

  1) Uterine cancer by 300%.
  2) Stroke by 43%.
  3) Pulmonary embolism by threefold.
  4) Uterine sarcoma.

Discussion

As noted in The Journal of Family Practice, "At best using Tamoxifen to treat 1000 high risk women for five years would prevent seventeen cases of invasive breast cancer and seven cases of noninvasive breast cancer, while contributing to at least seven uterine cancers and two pulmonary emboli." [1-3] Many women and their physicians have found the disadvantages of Tamoxifen including possible life-threatening uterine cancers, strokes, pulmonary embolisms and uterine sarcomas to be an unacceptable risk given the fact that at best Tamoxifen appears to reduce the risk of breast cancer by about 50% in women at high risk. Tamoxifen has no effect on women who develop estrogen receptor negative breast cancer and is not indicated in young women or women who are at low to moderate risk.

Raloxifene has been approved for the treatment of osteoporosis and there are several studies that show that it does reduce breast cancer risk for those women at high risk. Additionally, it does not appear to increase the risk of uterine cancer, as has been noted with Tamoxifen. The disadvantages still include an increased risk of deep vein blood clots (venous thrombosis) which have the possibility of developing into pulmonary emboli (blood clots that go to the lungs, which could be a life-threatening phenomenon). Raloxifene does not reduce postmenopausal symptoms; therefore many women continue to have hot flashes, night sweats, sleep disturbances, cognitive dysfunctions and other menopausal symptoms while on Raloxifene. For some women, Raloxifene made the hot flashes worse. (It should be noted that for most women this was a temporary phenomenon lasting for several months.) Raloxifene does appear to have a more benign side effect profile than Tamoxifen. That having been said, it still has increased risk of significant, possible life-threatening side effects including venous thrombosis. Therefore, it should be considered only for those women at a very high risk of breast cancer.

If you are at low to moderate risk for breast cancer, then you should institute the changes that we have reviewed in this book. At this point in time, the SERMS are not indicated for those of you in the low to moderate risk group. If you are in a high risk group, then certainly you should institute the changes we have discussed in this book first. There are several studies which indicate nutrients such as I3C/DIM, may actually improve the cancer prevention effect of the SERMS. The SERMS, however, are only indicated for five years of use, the longer you are on the SERMS the greater the apparent possibility of the side effects we have discussed. Many of my patients are very uncomfortable with SERMS and their possible side effects. I do not and have not prescribed the SERMS, but certainly I have seen many patients who are on the medications from their gynecologists. Whether or not to go on a SERM if you are at high risk is a difficult decision, one you must discuss very carefully with your gynecologist. I have very briefly discussed the advantages versus the disadvantages in this chapter for those of you who may not be familiar with these medications and for those of you who have had the SERMS presented to you as a treatment option, but may not be familiar with the down side of these medications. Unfortunately, it has been my clinical experience that in many cases the advantages have been explained to women in great detail and possibly even over emphasized and the disadvantages have been underemphasized.

---

[1] Physicians Desk Reference, 57th Edition (2003)
[2] "The Journal of Family Practice" (Dec 2001), Vol 30, No 12: p 1023
[3]Phillips O P M.D. "Raloxifene Versus Standard Hormone Replacement" The Female Patient, Vol 27 (May 2002)

21

Putting It All Together

What to do now.

EQ: Estrogen quotient

You must know your EQ! The 24 hour urine named the Estrogen Metabolism Evaluation will tell your EQ. Remember:

$$EQ = \frac{\text{Estriol } (E^3)}{\text{Estrone } (E^1) + \text{Estradiol } (E^2)}$$

If your EQ is less than 1.2:

(1) Consider changing your estrogen replacement therapy (ERT) to Estriol. (See Chapter 4)

(2) Add soy and flaxseed to your diet. (See Chapter 7)

EMI: Estrogen Metabolite Index.

You must know your EMI! Obtain this number from the 24 hour urine Estrogen Metabolism Evaluation (see above), or separately from the urine Estronex.™ (See Products/Services Chapter)

If Your EMI is Less Than 2:

(1) Increase the cruciferous vegetables in your diet. (See Chapter 5)

(2) Increase the soy and flaxseed in your diet. (See Chapter 7)

(3) Consider supplementation of bioavailable DIM or I3C. (See Chapter 6)

Repeat your EMI every 6 to 12 months until 2 or above.

Progesterone

You must know your progesterone! Obtain this through a saliva progesterone. (See Products/Services Section)

If your progesterone is low:

(1) Consider the addition of bio-identical progesterone cream. (See Chapter 9)

Bone Density

You must know your bone density! You can find this out by:

(1) Urine for bone loss markers. (See Products/Services Section)

(2) Dual Photon Densitometry: of lumbar spine, hip and wrist. (See your family doctor.)

If bone density is low, consider:

(1) 2000 mg per day of absorbable calcium.

(2) Vitamin D 400 IU daily.

(3) Progesterone, if your progesterone is low. (See Chapter 9)

(4) Increase the soy foods in your diet.

(5) Consider Black Cohosh or Estriol if not on estrogen replacement. (If you have menopausal symptoms.)

(6) Consider Calcitonin or Bisphosphonate (Fosamax™, Actonel™).

(7) Consider Boron and trace minerals.

(8) Repeat your urine for bone loss in 6 to 12 months and your densitometry as directed by your healthcare practitioner.

Antioxidants

If your B12 and folate levels are low (See Products/Services Section), consider:

(1) 1000 mcg B12 sublingual daily.

(2) Folate 1 mg daily.

To know your levels, have a blood B-12 and Folate done by your doctor (See Chapter 16), or urinary methylmalonate/methyl-tetrahydrofolate level completed. (See Product/Services Section)

Glutathione (GTH)

- Know your glutathione level or consider: N-acetyl-cysteine (NAC) 500 mg q.d. to help your body make GTH.
- Add as many fresh organic vegetables to your diet as possible.
- Add green tea and tumeric as often as possible and consider curcumin supplementation. (See Chapter 11 & 12)

Estrogen Detoxification

If your level of beta glucuronidase is elevated, consider adding calcium glucarate and a probiotic (good bacteria) supplement (See Products and Services Section). Your beta glucuronidase level can be determined by a special stool test (See Products and Services Section.) Along with beta glucuronidase, the complete digestive stool test will tell you if your bowel is overgrown with "bad" pathogenic bacteria or yeast. It will also give you the level of "good" bacteria.

Products/Services

Products available at Vital Health Center
www.vitalhealthcenter.com
Toll Free 1-888-244-3774

Estronex™
Urine test that will give your 20H/160H Ratio (EMI).

24° urine EMI plus EQ
More extensive urine study that will give your levels of Estriol E^3, Estradiol E^2, and Estrone E^1 (therefore your EQ), in addition to your EMI 20H/160H Ratio.

Urine for Bone Loss
This test will give you bone loss markers to help determine if you are actively losing bone.

Saliva Progesterone
This simple saliva test will give your level of free progesterone, which is the type available for use by the body. (If you are cycling, do this test on day 21 of your cycle.)

Urine for Organic Acids
This easy urine test will give your levels of folate, vitamin B12, sulfur (an important antioxidant) plus information on how well your metabolism is working (Krebs Cycle) AND indicators of overgrowth of abnormal bowel bacteria and/or yeast.

Complete Stool Analysis
This easy to complete stool test will give your B-glucurmadase levels plus levels of good bacteria versus pathogenic "bad" bacteria and/or yeast.

Vitality Today Monthly Newsletter
Dr. Edward J. Conley's cutting edge monthly e-newsletter designed to give you the information you need for optimal health.
***Subscribe through www.vitalhealthcenter.com**

Supplements

Supplements available at Vital Health Center
www.vitalhealthcenter.com
Toll Free 1-888-244-3774

Indole: Combination of I3C plus bioavailable DIM...

Vitamin E with mixed tocopherols..........................

Tocotrienols....... ....

Black Cohosh...

Super Curcumin...

Folate/B12 (Methylcobalamin)..........................

Absorbable calcium ....

MSM: organic form of sulfur, necessary for detoxification...

IP-6: Immune enhancer to improve Natural Killer Cell function...

Soy phytoestrogens......................................

Tea Polyphenols...

Antioxidant Complex...................................

Multi-Probiotic (good bacteria)........................

Theraslim™: natural starch blocker – weight loss product...

INDEX

A

B

F

G

H

I

K

L

M

N